PERIPHERAL NEUROPATHY - A NEW INSIGHT INTO THE MECHANISM, EVALUATION AND MANAGEMENT OF A COMPLEX DISORDER

Edited by **Nizar Souayah**

Peripheral Neuropathy - A New Insight into the Mechanism, Evaluation and Management of a Complex Disorder
http://dx.doi.org/10.5772/56421
Edited by Nizar Souayah

Contributors

Yuko Kanbayashi, Toyoshi Hosokawa, Lauren E. Ta, Emily Ramirez, Anthony Windebank, Charles Loprinzi, Kathrine Jáuregui-Renaud, Sabatino Maione, Enza Palazzo, Javier Lopez-Mendoza, Alexandro Aguilera Salgado, Chengyuan Li

Published by InTech

Janeza Trdine 9, 51000 Rijeka, Croatia

Copyright © 2013 InTech

Notice

Publishing Process Manager Ana Pantar
Technical Editor InTech DTP team
Cover InTech Design team

Additional hard copies can be obtained from orders@intechopen.com

Peripheral Neuropathy - A New Insight into the Mechanism, Evaluation and Management of a Complex Disorder, Edited by Nizar Souayah
p. cm.
ISBN 978-953-51-1060-6

For EU product safety concerns:
IN TECH d.o.o., Prolaz Marije Krucifikse Kozulić 3, 51000 Rijeka, Croatia,
info@intechopen.com or visit our website at intechopen.com.

Meet the editor

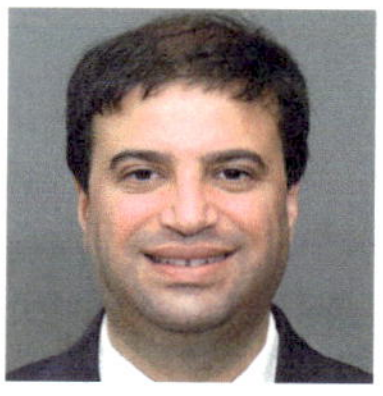

Dr Nizar Souayah is a neuromuscular program director and a faculty member at the University of Medicine and Dentistry of New Jersey. He is board certified in Neurology, Psychiatry and Neuromuscular Disorders from the American Board of Psychiatry and Neurology. He is also board certified in Electrodiagnostic Medicine from the American Board of Electrodiagnotic Medicine. He is an active member of the American Academy of Neurology and a fellow of the American Association of Neuromuscular & Electrodiagnostic Medicine. Dr Souayah published extensively in the field of Neurology. He published more than 180 peer reviewed manuscripts, abstracts, poster presentations and books in the neurology and neuromuscular disorders field, including the peripheral neuropathy field. He contributed to several national and international neuroscience meetings. He is also directing a basic sciences laboratory focusing on translational research in inflammatory and neurodegenerative disease.

Contents

Preface

Understanding the rapid changes in the evaluation and management of peripheral neuropathies, as well as the complexity of their mechanism, is a mandatory requirement for the practitioner to optimize patient's care. The objective of this book is to update health care professionals on recent advances in the pathogenesis, diagnosis and treatment of peripheral neuropathy. This work was written by a group of clinicians and scientists with large expertise in the field. In the first chapter of section one, Dr Emily A Ramirez and collaborators reviewed the pathogenesis of neuropathic pain and identified the anatomical pathways and the molecular mechanism of neuropathic pain. They reviewed the interaction between the central and peripheral nervous system in chronic pain as well as its clinical assessment and treatment. In the second chapter of section one, Dr Chengyuan Li and collaborators reviewed the pharmacological management of diabetic neuropathy. This was based on translational research from animal models of diabetic peripheral neuropathy. In the third chapter of section one, Dr Sabatino Maione and collaborators reviewed the complex mechanisms of painful neuropathy involving the central and peripheral nervous system. Based on these mechanisms, they evaluated the use of cannabinoids and stem cells for the treatment of peripheral neuropathy. Dr Mendoza and Dr Salgado reviewed the diagnosis and management of compressive neuropathies in the first chapter of section two. In the second chapter of this section, Dr Jáuregui-Renaud provided a comprehensive review on the role of Postural balance in the evaluation of peripheral neuropathy. In the last chapter of section two, Dr Kanbayashi and Dr Hosokawa reviewed the most recent advances in the pharmacotherapy of postherpetic neuralgia.

I dedicate this work to the memory of my father, for his enduring love and guidance throughout my career, he continued to serve as a source of inspiration. I extend my gratitude to my mother for her love and affection. I am continuously indebted to my wife Sonia for her love, unconditional support and encouragement, without her help and sacrifice, this work would not have been possible. I am also grateful to my son Sami and my beautiful daughters Leila and Nora for their love and energy which continue to be a valuable source of inspiration.

Dr Nizar Souayah
Neuromuscular Medicine Program Director
Director of Peripheral Neuropathy Center
Department of Neurology and Neuroscience
University of Medicine & Dentistry of New Jersey, USA

Section 1

Peripheral Neuropathy: From Bench to Bedside

Chapter 1

Neuropathic Pain: From Mechanism to Clinical Application

Emily A. Ramirez, Charles L. Loprinzi,
Anthony Windebank and Lauren E. Ta

Additional information is available at the end of the chapter

http://dx.doi.org/10.5772/55277

1. Introduction

A lesion or disease affecting the somatosensory system can cause a wide range of pathophysiologic symptoms including mild or severe chronic pain. Due to the diversity of etiologies giving rise to nervous system damage that generates neuropathic pain, it has become a ubiquitous health concern without respect for geographic or socioeconomic boundaries [1]. Within the developing world, infectious diseases [2-4] and trauma [5] are the most common sources of neuropathic pain syndromes. The developed world, in contrast, suffers more frequently from diabetic polyneuropathy (DPN) [6, 7], post herpetic neuralgia (PHN) from herpes zoster infections [8], and chemotherapy-induced peripheral neuropathy (CIPN) [9, 10]. There is relatively little epidemiological data regarding the prevalence of neuropathic pain within the general population, but a few estimates suggest it is around 7-8% [11, 12]. Despite the widespread occurrence of neuropathic pain, treatment options are limited and often ineffective, leaving many to live with the persistent agony and psychosocial burden associated with chronic pain [13, 14].

Neuropathic pain can present as on-going or spontaneous discomfort that occurs in the absence of any observable stimulus or a painful hypersensitivity to temperature and touch. This limits physical capabilities and impairs emotional well-being, often interfering with an individual's ability to earn a living or maintain healthy relationships. It is not surprising, therefore, that people with chronic pain have increased incidence of anxiety and depression and reduced scores in quantitative measures of health related quality of life [15].

Despite significant progress in chronic and neuropathic pain research, which has led to the discovery of several efficacious treatments in rodent models, pain management in humans remains ineffective and insufficient [16]. The lack of translational efficiency may be due to inadequate animal models that do not faithfully recapitulate human disease or from biological differences between rodents and humans [16]. Whatever the cause, the translational gap necessitates a bridge between clinicians and basic researchers in order to move from the clinic to the laboratory and back into the clinic.

In an attempt to increase the efficacy of medical treatment for neuropathic pain, clinicians and researchers have been moving away from an etiology based classification towards one that is mechanism based. It is current practice to diagnose a person who presents with neuropathic pain according to the underlying etiology and lesion topography [17]. However, this does not translate to effective patient care as these classification criteria do not suggest efficacious treatment. A more apt diagnosis might include a description of symptoms and the underlying pathophysiology associated with those symptoms. This chapter attempts to define neuropathic pain at the cellular and molecular level, as seen by a laboratory scientist, and then describe how the manifestations of these pathophysiologic changes are observed in the clinic, as seen by a clinician. It will then discuss a merger of the two points of view and suggest how this can lead to better patient care through more effective treatment.

2. Definition of neuropathic pain

Neuropathic pain has been defined by the International Association for the Study of Pain (IASP) as "pain arising as the direct consequence of a lesion or disease affecting the somatosensory system" [18]. This is distinct from nociceptive pain – which signals tissue damage through an intact nervous system – in underlying pathophysiology, severity, and associated psychological comorbidities [13]. Individuals who suffer from neuropathic pain syndromes report pain of higher intensity and duration than individuals with non-neuropathic chronic pain and have significantly increased incidence of depression, anxiety, and sleep disorders [13, 19].

Any trauma to the somatosensory system appears to have the capacity to cause a neuropathic pain syndrome; yet the presence of any individual pathology does not guarantee the development of neuropathic pain, highlighting the importance of genetic and environmental factors as well as individual disease pathogenesis. To further complicate matters, individuals with seemingly identical diseases who both develop neuropathic pain may experience distinct abnormal sensory phenotypes. This may include a loss of sensory perception in some modalities and increased activity in others. Often a reduction in the perception of vibration and light touch is coupled with positive sensory symptoms such as paresthesia, dysesthesia, and pain [20]. Pain may manifest as either spontaneous, with a burning or shock-like quality, or as a hypersensitivity to mechanical or thermal stimuli [21]. This hypersensitivity takes two forms: allodynia, pain that is evoked from a normally non-painful stimulus, and hyperalgesia, an exaggerated pain response from a moderately painful stimulus. For a more extensive list of sensory signs and symptoms associated with neuropathic pain see Table 1. Ultimately, the path towards efficacious treatment of chronic pain will include a clear understanding of how certain pathophysiologic changes lead to specific sensory signs and symptoms. This will allow clinicians to translate measurable sensory abnormalities into underlying pathology. With a clear view of mechanism, targeted treatment and individualized medicine become conceivable.

3. Anatomical overview of pain as a somatosensory modality

At the turn of the 20th century Charles Sherrington proposed the concept of pain-specific neural circuitry and deemed neurons within this circuit "nociceptors" [22]. This "specificity theory" of pain was competing for favor with the prevailing "pattern theory" which held that pain was encoded by the same low-threshold sensory nerve endings that transmit information about vibration and light touch through high frequency stimulation and central summation [23]. It is now clear, as Sherrington proposed that the sensation of pain is encoded by a unique set of peripheral and central neurons whose primary purpose is to alert the organism to a potentially dangerous situation.

The nociceptive system detects noxious stimuli (i.e. that are of a sufficient magnitude to cause bodily injury) and elicits appropriate avoidance behaviors. Detection begins with free nerve endings in the skin or viscera that carry specialized membrane receptors capable of converting high magnitude chemical, mechanical, or thermal energy into an electrical impulse. The impulse is carried from the periphery to the dorsal horn of the spinal cord where neurotransmitter release relays the activity to second order neurons. Here, signals from the periphery are integrated with information from descending sources that modulate nociceptive circuitry in a manner that is dependent on the environmental context. The sum of this exchange is carried by secondary projection neurons to supraspinal nuclei which interpret the signal and create the conscious perception of pain.

The nociceptive circuit is not static, however; there is tremendous plasticity, from the periphery to the neocortex, which modulates the perception of pain to reflect the physiological needs of the organism and optimize survival. This is best understood by considering two examples of hypo- and hyper- sensitivity to pain: a time of war and an illness, respectively. Perceiving pain during a period of intense stress, such as wartime, would decrease chances of survival by increasing vulnerability to a more immediate threat. Conversely, in a low stress environment activation of the inflammatory response as a result of illness or injury sensitizes nociceptors leading to pain hypersensitivity, rest, and healing. Neuropathic pain, therefore, can be considered an inappropriate hijacking of inherent neuronal plasticity to promote hypersensitivity in contexts where it is not beneficial.

4. Peripheral nociceptors detect a noxious stimulus

Noxious stimuli are perceived by small diameter peripheral neurons whose free nerve endings are distributed throughout the body. These neurons are distinct from, although anatomically proximal to, the low threshold mechanoreceptors responsible for the perception of vibration and light touch. Both low and high threshold afferents are pseudounipolar neurons of the dorsal root and trigeminal ganglion with peripheral terminals that extend into the skin/viscera and central terminals that extend into the gray matter of the spinal cord or trigeminal nucleus caudalis depending on whether they originated from the body or face, respectively. Low threshold afferents, or Aβ fibers, can be distinguished from nociceptors by biochemical and electrophysiological properties. Aβ neurons are large diameter, heavily myelinated, and fast conducting fibers, while nociceptors fall into one of two functionally distinct categories: lightly myelinated, medium diameter (1-5 μm) Aδ fibers that mediate a sharp, well localized "first" pain and unmyelinated, small diameter (0.2 – 1.5μm) C fibers that mediate a duller, anatomically diffuse "second" pain. Together with Aα fibers (which will not be considered here) Aβ, Aδ, and C fibers constitute the somatosensory system.

5. Membrane receptors capture energy and modulate excitability

As mentioned above, the purpose of these primary afferents is to detect noxious stimuli in the environment, for example a hot stove, or within the body as in an acidic or chemically unbalanced stomach. This requires the translation of chemical or high magnitude mechanical and thermal energy into an electrical impulse, a function carried out by a myriad of specialized receptors and ion channels (e.g. sodium and potassium channels, G-coupled protein receptors, receptor tyrosine kinases) that are embedded in the neuronal membrane. In addition to primary detection of the stimulus, these specialized receptors/ion channels also play an important role in nociceptive plasticity by regulating membrane excitability and dictating the magnitude of stimulus required to generate an action potential.

A major breakthrough in understanding how nociceptors detect environmental stimuli came with the discovery of the transient receptor potential (TRP) family of nonselective cation channels [24]. These membrane-bound receptors – for the first time – provided a substrate by which noxious energy could elicit neuronal depolarization. Each of the twenty-eight known TRP family members has a unique profile of activation that includes thermal and chemical stimuli [25]. The most well-characterized TRP channel, TRPV1, is activated by temperatures >42°C and the chemical compound capsaicin (the "hot" component of chili peppers) under normal physiological conditions [24]. In pathological states, TRPV1 has been implicated in pain hypersensitivity in models of inflammation, diabetic neuropathy [26, 27], partial nerve injury [28, 29], and chemotherapy- induced painful neuropathy [30]. Mechanistically, TRPV1 mediated hypersensitivity occurs as the result of changes in the expression, trafficking, and activation potential of TRPV1 following nerve injury [31]. Components of the inflammatory soup can modify TRPV1 by either direct allosteric modulation or indirect modification. For example, protons may bind directly to the extracellular domain, or stimulation of membrane bound receptor tyrosine kinases may trigger intracellular signaling cascades that result in phosphorylation of an intracellular domain. These physical modifications lead to altered activation kinetics and ultimately a lowered thermal or mechanical threshold for individual nociceptors (Figure 1) [31]. The behavioral correlate of a cellular lowering of threshold is hypersensitivity to thermal or mechanical stimuli i.e. allodynia and hyperalgesia.

http://dx.doi.org/10.5772/55277

In addition to hypersensitivity, individuals with neuropathic pain frequently experience ongoing spontaneous pain as a major source of discomfort and distress. Following trauma to the peripheral nerve, ectopic activity was observed in primary nociceptors in the periphery, suggesting this to be the major source of spontaneous pain [32]. In healthy individuals, a quiescent neuron will only generate an action potential when presented with a stimulus of sufficient magnitude to cause membrane depolarization. Following nerve injury, however, significant changes in ion channel expression, distribution, and kinetics lead to disruption of the homeostatic electric potential of the membrane resulting in oscillations and burst firing. This manifests as spontaneous pain that has a shooting or burning quality [31]. Three types of ion channels seem to mediate this effect: two-pore domain K^+ channels (TRESK and TREK-2), voltage gated sodium channels (VGSC; i.e. $Na_v1.8$, $Na_v1.6$, $Na_v1.1$, $Na_v1.9$) and hyperpolarization-activated cyclic nucleotide-gated (HCN) channels (Figure 1) [31]. There is reasonable evidence to suggest that individual ion channels contribute to specific neuropathic pain symptoms; for example $Na_v1.8$ plays a role in cold-induced allodynia (for review see [33, 34]). The exact nature and extent of this relationship is unclear, but it provides an intriguing therapeutic possibility: unambiguous pharmacologic ion channel blockers to relieve individual sensory symptoms with minimal unintended effects allowing pain relief without global numbness.

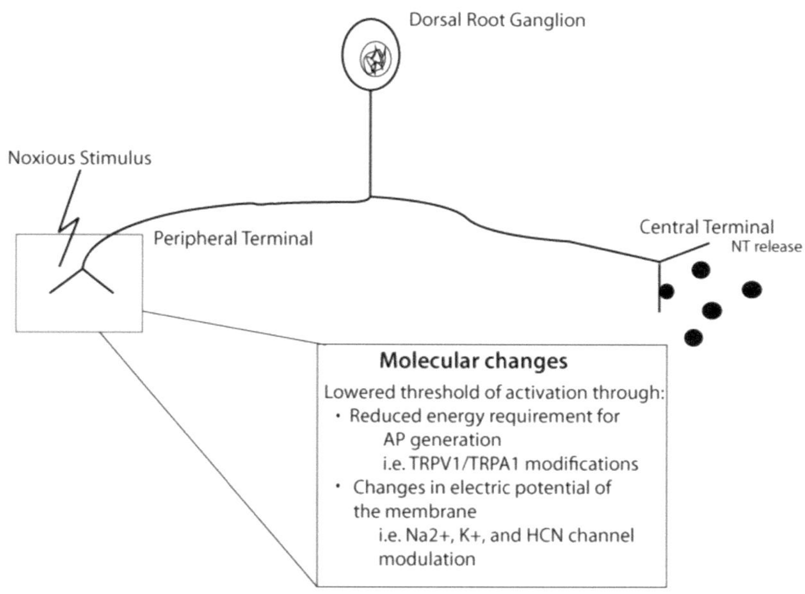

Figure 1. Pathophysiological changes associated with a primary afferent nociceptor. A pseudounipolar C-fiber detects a stimulus in the skin or viscera, and an action potential (AP) is propagated along the axon prompting neurotransmitter (NT) release from the central terminal. Following nerve injury, modulation and modification of molecular components can lead to painful hypersensitivity to stimuli as well as spontaneous or ongoing pain. For simplification we portray a unidirectional flow of information, but it's interesting to note that generation of an AP or NT release as well as the associated pathophysiological changes can occur at either terminal.

6. Pain circuits of the dorsal horn integrate information

A cross section of a spinal cord reveals morphologically and biochemically distinct layers of gray matter – Laminae of Rexed after the scientist who first described them – that integrate input from a variety of ascending and descending sources (Figure 2) [35]. Each layer forms a functional compartment containing a dense network of primary afferents, secondary projection neurons, descending fibers, and interneurons with unique patterns of connectivity. The most superficial layers of the dorsal horn, laminae I and II, receive peripheral input almost exclusively from Aδ and C fibers while Aβ fibers innervate more medial laminae (III-IV)[36]. Lamina V contains wide dynamic range polymodal projection neurons that receive direct input from Aδ and Aβ fibers as well as indirect input from C fibers [36]. Thus, it appears there is both anatomical segregation (laminae I-IV) and integration (laminae V) of painful and non-painful stimuli at the level of the spinal cord, providing the substrate for distinct pathophysiological mechanisms in the development of neuropathic pain.

It should be noted that primary afferents originating from the orofacial region project to the trigeminal nucleus caudalis of the medulla rather than the dorsal horn of the spinal cord [37]. Similar organization, function, and pathophysiological mechanisms are observed in both nuclei, so they will not be considered separately.

7. Central sensitization leads to painful hypersensitivity

Functional and structural changes of dorsal horn circuitry lead to pain hypersensitivity that is maintained independent of peripheral sensitization [38]. This central sensitization provides a mechanistic explanation for the sensory abnormalities that occur in both acute and chronic pain states, such as the expansion of hypersensitivity beyond the innervation territory of a lesion site, repeated stimulation of a constant magnitude leading to an increasing pain response, and pain outlasting a peripheral stimulus [39-41]. In healthy individuals, acute pain triggers central sensitization, but homeostatic sensitivity returns following clearance of the initial insult. In some individuals who develop neuropathic pain, genotype and environmental factors contribute to maintenance of central sensitization leading to spontaneous pain, hyperalgesia, and allodynia.

At the cellular level, potentiation or facilitation of synapses in the dorsal horn leads to central sensitization. The former is a type of homosynaptic strengthening whereby repeated neurotransmitter release from a primary nociceptor leads to post-synaptic molecular remodeling in second order neurons, ultimately reducing the quantity of neurotransmitter required to generate an action potential (i.e. hyperalgesia). This process resembles long term potentiation (LTP), the molecular correlate of learning and memory, differing in the time-scale of associated post-synaptic changes and several molecular components [42]. Like LTP, potentiation of nociceptors in the dorsal horn is dependent on the post-synaptic function of ionotropic glutamate receptors (N-Methyl-D-aspartic acid receptors; NMDAR) suggesting that this may be a viable target for treating centrally maintained neuropathic pain.

http://dx.doi.org/10.5772/55277

Similarly, facilitation also results in a lowered activation threshold in second order neurons, but distinct from potentiation, the molecular changes occur in a nearby dendritic spine rather than the spine receiving the nociceptive input. If the nearby dendritic spine is a silent partner of an Aβ afferent, molecular changes that lower the threshold recruit this primary afferent into nociceptive circuitry resulting in the perception of pain from innocuous stimuli (i.e. allodynia).

In addition to heterosynaptic strengthening, phenotypic changes or dendritic sprouting of Aβ fibers can lead to the incorporation of low threshold mechanoreceptors into pain circuitry.

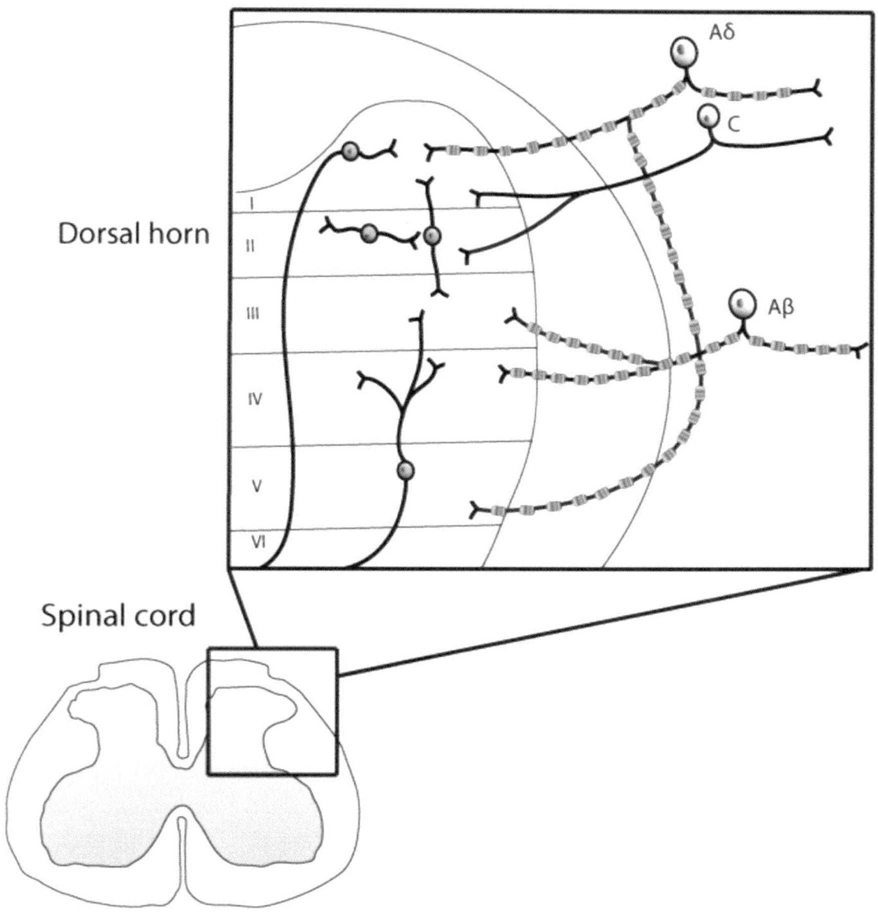

Figure 2. Neuronal architecture of the dorsal horn. Laminae (represented by numerals I-VI) are morphologically and functionally distinct layers within the gray matter of the spinal cord. Lamina I primarily contains large projection neurons that send processes up the spinal cord towards higher brain regions. Lamina II, in contrast, is more heavily populated with interneurons, many of which supply inhibitory signals to lamina I projection neurons. Lamina V contains wide dynamic range neurons that receive primary input from multiple sensory modalities. Peripheral afferents project to distinct laminae. While Aδ and C fibers are associated with superficial laminae, Aβ fibers project more medially. For a comprehensive review of dorsal horn circuitry see [36].

Two neuropeptides, substance P (SP) and calcitonin gene-related peptide (CGRP) are normally exclusively expressed by Aδ and C fibers in the periphery. Following nerve injury, however, Aβ fibers begin to manufacture these neuropeptides [43]. Additionally, there is evidence to suggest that remodeling of Aβ dendritic arbors can create novel circuitry [44]. These changes all manifest as dynamic mechanical allodynia.

In contrast to the gain-of-function changes that take place in Aβ fibers following injury, inhibitory descending and interneurons experience a sharp loss-of-function. This loss of inhibitory input releases the brake on neurotransmission and increases the excitatory current in the superficial dorsal horn [45]. Although there is evidence that excitotoxicity contributes to apoptotic loss of gamma-amino butyric acid (GABA)-ergic interneurons and descending inhibitory neurons of the rostroventral medulla [46, 47], it has been argued that injury-induced disinhibition is the result of attenuated efficacy of intact GABAergic interneurons that occurs independent of cell death [48-50]. Activation of microglia, resident macrophages of the nervous system, is a pathological hallmark of nervous system damage [51]. Release of brain-derived neurotrophic factor (BDNF) from activated microglia is necessary and sufficient to shift the anion reversal potential in lamina I projection neurons, reducing the effect of GABA in these neurons [52]. Specifically targeting BDNF or activated microglia may be a viable treatment for neuropathic pain.

8. Supraspinal nuclei interpret the signal

Activation of peripheral nociceptors elicits a complex behavioral response that allows an organism to avoid the noxious stimulus immediately (by moving away from the source) and in the future (by enhanced learning and memory). To carry out the sum of these behaviors the pain circuit recruits a large number of cortical and subcortical regions that manage a variety of aspects of cognition and perception. Prominent examples include areas of the brain associated with motivation/reward, learning/memory, and somatosensation (reviewed in [53]). Classically, pain in the brain has been described in terms of a particular pattern of activation referred to as the "pain matrix". Areas of the matrix can be classified as belonging to one of two parallel pathways that control distinct aspects of pain: sensory discrimination (e.g. location, duration, and intensity) or affective/motivational (e.g. feelings of suffering and avoidance behaviors) [54, 55]. Increasing evidence gathered from rapidly evolving technology has suggested this description to be an oversimplification, however, as it applies uniquely to healthy individuals with experimentally induced acute pain [53]. Although useful, it is important for the future of pain research and treatment that we continue evaluate the current schematic, employing new technologies as they develop.

9. Decoding pain representation in the brain

Recent progress has expanded the current view of pain representation and encoding in the brain by utilizing functional magnetic resonance imaging (fMRI), MR spectroscopy, MR morphometry, and diffusion tensor MRI. In a comprehensive review, Apkarian and colleagues summarize this recent progress and propose a model that includes a temporal, as well as a spatial, cerebral representation of pain [53]. They've suggested that in the context of acute thermal pain activity in the anterior insula, nucleus accumbens (NAc), and mid-cingulum peak prior to the conscious perception of pain, the "anticipation", while perception is distinctly correlated with peak activity in the anterior cingulate, mid- and posterior insula, and portions of the dorsal striatum. Lastly, as the stimulus is extinguished bringing about "relief" regions of the brainstem, in particular the periaqueductal grey (PAG), become active [53].

Another significant finding led to the disentanglement of the neural coding for two distinct dimensions of a stimulus: the objective magnitude of an applied stimulus and an individual's subjective perception of stimulus intensity. Again using fMRI in the context of acute thermal pain, Baliki et. al. suggest that actual stimulus intensity is encoded by large portions of the cingulate and insular cortices while specific subsections of each, namely the anterior portion of the cingulate and the posterior insula, correlate strongly with subjective perception [56]. Thus it appears that pain perception follows a similar processing stream as other sensory modalities (e.g. vision, hearing, olfaction) wherein information about subjective magnitude is extracted by specific regions of the insular cortex [53]. These findings are beginning to lay the foundation for a clear and accurate representation of spatiotemporal coding of pain in the brain, with the ultimate goal of correlating neural activity with distinct cognitive and behavioral functions.

10. Morphological and functional changes in the brain are associated with chronic pain

Chronic pain conditions are associated with vast functional and structural changes of the brain, when compared to healthy controls, but it is currently unclear which comes first: does chronic pain cause distortions of brain circuitry and anatomy or do cerebral abnormalities trigger and/or maintain the perception of chronic pain? Future studies will clarify these questions.

Brain abnormalities in chronic pain states include modification of brain activity patterns, localized decreases in gray matter volume, and circuitry rerouting [53]. Observation of overall brain activity patterns in a variety of chronic pain conditions has led to the discovery that spontaneous and evoked pain are uniquely represented in the brain [53]. Spontaneous pain associated with chronic back pain and PHN induce increased activity in the mPFC and amygdale while acute thermal pain and allodynia associated with PHN illicit larger responses in the thalamus and insula [53]. Similar activity patterns are observed in thermal and mechanical acute pain in healthy individuals and knee pain associated with osteoarthritis, all forms of evoked pain [53].

Chronic pain conditions are associated with localized reduction in gray matter volume, and the topography of gray matter volume reduction is dictated, at least in part, by the particular pathology. Chronic back pain, for example, is associated with a loss of bilateral dorsolateral prefrontal cortex and unilateral thalamic gray matter [57] while irritable bowel syndrome displays a volume reduction in the insula and cingulate cortex [58]. In addition, gray matter atrophy has been suggested to occur in a variety of pain conditions including fibromyalgia, knee osteoarthritis, and headaches [59-66]. These changes appear to represent a form of plasticity as they are reversible when pain is effectively managed [63, 67, 68]. How or why individual pathologies result in distinct morphological distortions and what impact these changes have on individual pain perception remains to be determined.

Changes in brain circuitry have also been reported in patients with chronic back pain [69]. Baliki et. al. found that when an acute thermal stimulus is applied to the skin of healthy subjects, activity in the NAc at the end of the stimulus response cycle is strongly correlated with the insula. This is distinct from patients with chronic back pain where activity in the NAc is strongly correlated with the medial prefrontal cortex (mPFC) [69]. The resulting activity in the NAc is divergent as the phasic response observed in healthy subjects has been correlated to the prediction of reward while the activity pattern in chronic pain patients represents lack of reward or disappointment [69]. Although there is no difference in the reported perceived magnitude of the stimulus, this suggests that subconsciously chronic pain patients are disappointed when an acute pain stimulus is removed, begging the question, what are the resultant cognitive and behavior manifestations? This opens up the field to a series of questions considering the effects of subconscious components of brain activity on perception of pain and resultant behaviors.

11. Neuropathic pain diagnosis

Persistent pain is the single most common ailment that brings people to a primary care physician each year, accounting for approximately 40% of all visits [70]. Measurements of overall health-related quality of life, a multidimensional construct that takes into account physical, emotional, and social well-being, are depressed in chronic pain patients [15], and the resulting work absenteeism and elevated health care costs represent a substantial economical and societal burden [71-74]. Although effective management of chronic pain would certainly reduce this burden, treatment options are inadequate and often wrought with adverse health effects [15]. It is becoming increasingly clear that the path towards efficacious pain management is one of individualized medicine that stems from an understanding of the underlying pathophysiology and resultant sensory abnormalities [31, 75-77]. Although this may be the future of pain management, the current understanding of an individual "sensory phenotype" and dearth of clinical trials utilizing this perspective prevent immediate implementation. The following sections will highlight the current evidence based methods of diagnosing and treating neuropathic pain and suggest the future of research and clinical practice.

12. Clinical history

By definition, neuropathic pain indicates direct pathology of the nervous system while nociceptive pain is an indication of real or potential tissue damage. Due to the distinction in pathophysiology, conventional treatments prescribed for nociceptive pain are not very effective in treating neuropathic pain and vice versa [78]. Therefore the first step towards meaningful pain relief is an accurate diagnosis.

Identifying neuropathic pain in a clinical setting begins with a thorough review of the patient's history through evaluation of previous medical records and verbal communication with the patient. Standardized screening tools such as the Leeds Assessment of Neuropathic Symptoms and Signs (LANSS) [79], the Douleur Neuropathique en 4 questions (DN4) [12], and painDE-TECT [13] can guide clinician through a series of questions aimed at indentifying possible neuropathic pain. In completing these questionnaires patients are asked to describe their pain in terms of quality (i.e. pricking, tingling, pins and needles, electric shocks/shooting, burning) and context (i.e. provoked by heat, cold, or pressure) [80]. In addition to verbal descriptors, the LANSS and DN4 also include a short bedside examination of sensory abnormalities. Although each screening tool is unique, they have similar sensitivity and specificity, between 80-85% for both parameters [80]. This suggests that approximately 1 in 5 patients who fit the criteria for neuropathic pain as determined by the screening tool and 20% of all individuals who've been evaluated are misdiagnosed. This reaffirms that careful clinical judgment is necessary to make an accurate diagnosis.

Additional information that is not included within the standardized questionnaires can also be useful in diagnosing neuropathic pain. Mapping pain topography allows the clinician to consider whether a lesion is anatomically logical, and descriptions of frequency (i.e. on-going, spontaneous) and intensity (e.g. mild, moderate, severe, excruciating or 1-10) can aid in identifying a potential mechanism [1].

13. Clinical examination

Evaluating sensory function in a bedside examination can be helpful in assessing neuropathic pain. Since a lesion of the nervous system will often manifest as decreased sensitivity in some sensory modalities and increased sensitivity in others, objectively measuring each sensory modality can aid in forming a diagnosis. Guided by the patient's history, the putative lesion innervation territory is tested while the contralateral side of the body serves as a control. Testing consists of touching the patient's skin with calibrated tools that elicit a response in a subset of peripheral neurons. For example, brushing the skin lightly will tests sensitivity of Aβ mechanoreceptors while a thermoroller will test heat sensitive C fibers [1]. For a list of bedside sensory tests see Table 1.

14. Pharmacological treatment of neuropathic pain

Treating neuropathic pain requires a multifaceted approach that aims to eliminate the underlying etiology, when possible, and manage the associated discomforts and emotional distress. Although in some cases it is possible to directly treat the cause of neuropathic pain, for example surgery to alleviate a constricted nerve, it is more likely that the primary cause is untreatable, as is the case with singular traumatic events such as stroke and spinal cord injury and diseases like diabetes. When this is the case, symptom management and pain reduction become the primary focus. Unfortunately, in most cases complete elimination of pain is not a feasible endpoint; a pain reduction of 30% is considered to be efficacious [21]. Additionally, many pharmacological treatments require careful titration and tapering to prevent adverse effects and toxicity. This process may take several weeks to months, and ultimately the drug may be ineffective, necessitating another trial with a different medication. It is therefore necessary that both doctor and patient begin treatment with realistic expectations and goals.

Signs and Symptoms	Bedside Test	Pathological Response
Abnormal Sensations		
Hypoesthesia	Touch skin with cotton swab or gauze	Reduced sensation
Hypoalgesia	Prick skin with pin	Reduced sensation
Paraesthesia	Reported – grade intensity 1-10	
Spontaneous Pain		
Shooting	Reported – grade intensity 1-10	
Ongoing	Reported – grade intensity 1-10	
Evoked Pain		
Allodynia/Hyperalgesia		
Cold	Touch skin object <20°C	Painful, burning sensation
Heat	Touch skin object "/>40°C	Painful, burning sensation
Dynamic Mechanical	Move object (cotton swab or gauze) along skin	Sharp burning superficial pain in putative lesion territory as well as unaffected area
Punctate Mechanical	Pinprick with sharp object	Sharp burning superficial pain in putative lesion territory as well as unaffected area
Static Mechanical	Apply gentle pressure to skin	Dull pain in putative lesion territory as well as unaffected area
Temporal Summation	Pinprick with sharp object at 3s intervals for 30s	Sharp pain with increasing intensity

Table 1. A list of bedside tests used to identify signs and symptoms that are suggestive of neuropathic pain.

Recently, the Neuropathic Pain Special Interest Group (NeuPSIG) of the International Association for the Study of Pain reviewed the evidence–based guidelines for the pharmacological treatment of neuropathic pain and made recommendations that take into account clinical efficacy, adverse effects, effects on health related quality of life, convenience, and cost [81]. These findings as well as more recent evidence are reviewed here.

First-line medications for the treatment of neuropathic pain are those that have proven efficacy in randomized clinical trials (RCTs) and are consistent with pooled clinical observations [81]. These include antidepressants, calcium channel ligands, and topical lidocaine [15]. Tricyclic antidepressants (TCAs) have demonstrated efficacy in treating neuropathic pain with positive results in RCTs for central post-stroke pain, PHN, painful diabetic and non-diabetic polyneuropathy, and post-mastectomy pain syndrome [82]. However they do not seem to be effective in treating painful HIV-neuropathy or CIPN [82]. Duloxetine and venlafaxine, two selective serotonin norepinephrine reuptake inhibitors (SSNRIs), have been found to be effective in DPN and both DPN and painful polyneuropathies, respectively [81]. Adverse affects associated with TCAs and SSNRIs are relatively mild and can be mitigated by a slow titration beginning with a low dose [81].

Gabapentin and pregabalin have also demonstrated efficacy in several neuropathic pain conditions including DPN and PHN [81, 82]. Both drugs exert their effects by inhibiting neurotransmitter release through binding of the α_2-δ subunit of presynaptic calcium channels [83]. Adverse effects and efficacy of gabapentin and pregabalin are similar; however pregabalin may provide more rapid analgesia due to straightforward dosing determined by linear pharmacokinetic [78]. Topical lidocaine (5% patch or gel) has significantly reduced allodynia associated with PHN and other neuropathic pain syndromes in several RCTs [81, 82]. With no reported systemic adverse effects and mild skin irritation as the only concern, lidocaine is an appropriate choice for treating localized peripheral neuropathic pain.

In the event that first line medications, alone or in combination, are not effective at achieving adequate pain relief, second line medications may be considered. These include opioid analgesics and tramadol, pharmaceuticals which have proven efficacy in RCTs but are associated with significant adverse effects that warrant cautious prescription [15]. Although opioid analgesics are effective pain relievers in several types of neuropathic pain [81, 82, 84], they are associated with misuse or abuse, hypogonadism, constipation, nausea, and immunological changes [15]. Because many of these side effects can be mitigated by a low dose, careful titration, and short term use, opiates are an appropriate choice for treating acute or episodic neuropathic pain [81]. Careful consideration should be given when prescribing opiates to patients who have a personal or family history of drug or alcohol abuse, and additional monitoring to ensure appropriate use may be necessary.

Tramadol, a weak opioid μ-receptor agonist and serotonin and norepinephrine reuptake inhibitor (SNRI), is more effective than placebo but less effective than strong opioid μ-receptor agonists (e.g. morphine and oxycodone) in treating neuropathic pain [82]. Although the risk is considerably less than opioid analgesics, tramadol is also associated with abuse [81]. A rare but potentially fatal serotonin syndrome has been described, and tramadol may increase the likelihood of seizures or interact with other medications [15].

Recent clinical trials have considered additional intervention strategies with possible utility in treating neuropathic pain, although their efficacy remains to be determined. Treatments include botulinum toxin for PHN and postoperative allodynia [85, 86], high concentration capsaisin patch for the treatment of PHN and painful HIV neuropathy [15], and lacosamide, an antiepileptic drug with suggested efficacy in treating DPN [87-89]. There is also accumulating evidence that intravenous Ca^{2+} and Mg^{2+} may be effective at preventing CIPN caused a commonly used chemotherapeutic, oxaliplatin, without attenuating its antineoplastic efficacy [9].

15. Non-pharmacological treatment of neuropathic pain

The use of alternative and complementary medicine is on the rise, particularly in the United States [90]. Although anecdotal evidence abounds, there are relatively few RCTs supporting the use of such therapies. It is important in considering these treatments, however, that the lack of evidence is not read as evidence of lacking efficacy. The scarcity of well controlled, robust clinical trials considering non-pharmacological treatments of chronic pain makes it difficult to recommend or dismiss these alternative treatments. A few studies have examined the use of acupuncture, herbal therapy, massage, hypnosis, and biofeedback on easing chronic pain but have yielded mixed results (for a review see [90]). The difficulty in standardizing treatment, inherent to these multi-faceted approaches, is a major obstacle in drawing reliable conclusions. Additionally, small sample sizes and lack of obvious controls are also significant barriers. Despite these hurdles, which obscure evidence-based conclusions, non-pharmacological treatments are often prescribed in conjunction with evidence-based recommendations due to low risk of accompanying adverse effects.

Deep brain stimulation, a neurosurgical technique by which an implanted electrode delivers controlled electrical impulses to targeted brain regions, has demonstrated some efficacy in treating chronic pain but is not routinely employed due to a high risk-to-benefit ratio [91]. Targeting the periventricular/periaqueductal gray, internal capsule, and sensory thalamus has demonstrated efficacy in various pain conditions [91], but not all types of chronic pain are responsive. An intriguing new target, the NAc, has recently emerged as a potential site for deep brain stimulation as it has demonstrated efficacy in a case study of post-stroke pain [92]. As studies of pain processing in the brain have suggested, the pattern of activity in the NAc is divergent in nociceptive and chronic pain representation, validating this structure as a possible therapeutic target [69].

Another type of electro-stimulation device is emerging as a promising therapeutic tool for the treatment of neuropathic pain [93, 94]. Delivering repeated pulses of electrical stimulation trans-cutaneously, termed Scrambler therapy, has demonstrated some efficacy with lasting effects in CIPN [94], postsurgical pain, PHN, and spinal canal stenosis [93]. With few adverse effects and low associated risk, this may be a viable alternative to pharmacological treatment.

16. The future of neuropathic pain management correlating symptoms to mechanism

Limited efficacy of current pain treatment options has necessitated a revaluation of the standard classification of neuropathic pain in clinical practice [17] [31, 75-77]. It has been suggested that within etiology based neuropathic pain syndromes there are distinct subgroups

http://dx.doi.org/10.5772/55277

of patients who experience similar "symptom constellations" representing distinct pathophysiological mechanisms [95]. Furthermore, these symptom constellations can be seen, albeit in different proportions, across neuropathic pain syndromes, suggesting that the same underlying mechanism can cause neuropathic pain within and apart from the initiating etiology. Hypothetically, with this understanding comes an approach of targeted treatment that aims to identify the pathophysiological mechanism and specifically inhibit, block, or enhance the offending molecules. To implement this type of treatment will require a more intimate understanding of the mechanisms of neuropathic pain and the corresponding symptom manifestations. As this becomes defined, specific treatments can begin to emerge, and clinical trials can test the efficacy of this approach. See Table 2 for examples.

Signs and Symptoms	Example Mechanisms	Targeted Treatment
Spontaneous Pain		
Shooting	Ectopic impulse generation, Na^{2+} channel dysregulation	Selective Na^{2+} channel blocker
Ongoing	Inflammation in nerve root, central sensitization (potentiation), disinhibition	Cytokine antagonists, Calcium channel blocker, NMDA receptor antagonist
Evoked Pain		
Allodynia/Hyperalgesia		
Cold	Modulation of TRPM8 or Na^{2+} channels in peripheral nociceptors	TRPM8 receptor antagonist, Selective Na^{2+} channel blocker
Heat	Modulation of TRPV1 in peripheral nociceptors	TRPV1 receptor antagonist
Dynamic Mechanical	Central sensitization (potentiation and facilitation), disinhibition	Ca^{2+} channel blocker, NMDA receptor antagonist
Punctate Mechanical	Central sensitization (potentiation and facilitation), disinhibition	Ca^{2+} channel blocker, NMDA receptor antagonist
Static Mechanical	Modulation of unknown mechanoreceptors in peripheral nociceptors, TRPA1	?
Temporal Summation	Central sensitization	Ca^{2+} channel blocker, NMDA receptor antagonist

Table 2. Hypothetical examples of how signs and symptoms obtained in a bedside examination might indicate underlying pathophysiological mechanism. Once a putative mechanism has been established there is a potential for selective and specifically targeted treatments to be applied. For a comprehensive review see [21].

17. Genetic and environmental determinants of pain susceptibility

A major challenge in treating neuropathic pain is the heterogeneity of disease pathogenesis within an individual etiological classification. Patients with seemingly identical diseases may experience completely different neuropathic pain phenotypes, possibly due to genetic and environmental variation. A holistic approach to treating neuropathic pain, therefore, will require identification of risk or determinant factors that may play a role in neuropathic pain severity, progression, duration, or presentation.

Although there are major obstacles to studying the genetics of pain in humans, a few potential biomarkers have been identified [96]. A candidate gene association study, which compares allele frequencies between cohorts of patients with and without a particular trait, has yielded evidence that a polymorphism in catechol-O-methyltransferase (COMT) is associated with temporomandibular joint disorder [97, 98]. Other similar studies have identified alleles for the μ-opioid receptor 1 (OPRM1) [99] and the melanocortin-1 receptor (MCR1) [100] as potential determinants of sensitivity to opioid induced analgesia. A separate approach to identifying genetic determinants of pain biology uses rodent models and has also yielded promising results. Using this method, Tegeder et. al. identified a haplotype for the enzyme GTP cyclo-hydrolase 1 (GCH1), the rate limiting enzyme in the synthesis of tetrahydrobiopterin (BH4) [101]. BH4 is an important cofactor in the synthesis of serotonin, catecholamines, and all nitric oxide synthases [101] and plays a role in the development of chronic pain [96].

18. Conclusion

Neuropathic pain is a major source of physical and mental disability worldwide. It is associated with severe societal and individual psychosocial burden and will continue to be a major health concern until more effective treatments emerge. One of the biggest barriers to successful management of neuropathic pain has been the lack of understanding in the underlying pathophysiology that produces a pain phenotype. To that end, significant progress has been made in basic science research. From the discovery of the nociceptor and individual ion channel transducers to the mapping of pain representation in the brain, a foundational understanding has been laid. As we continue to build on this foundation, it is essential that strong communication exists between the laboratory and the clinic in order to ensure effective translation. With optimism we suggest that this could lead to better patient care and lessen the worldwide impact of neuropathic pain.

Acknowledgements

The authors are supported by National Institutes of Health grants NIDCR-DE020868 (LET), NCI-CA37404 (CLL and LET), and American Cancer Society- New Investigator Award (LET). We would like to thank Maja Radulovic for assistance in creating the figures.

http://dx.doi.org/10.5772/55277

Author details

Emily A. Ramirez[1], Charles L. Loprinzi[2], Anthony Windebank[1,3,4] and Lauren E. Ta[1,3,4*]

*Address all correspondence to: Ta.lauren@mayo.edu

1 Molecular Neuroscience Program, Graduate School, Mayo Clinic, College of Medicine, Rochester, Minnesota, USA

2 Division of Medical Oncology, Mayo Clinic, College of Medicine, Rochester, Minnesota, USA

3 Department of Neurology, Mayo Clinic, College of Medicine, Rochester, Minnesota, USA

4 Department of Neuroscience, Mayo Clinic, College of Medicine, Rochester, Minnesota, USA

References

[1] Haanpaa, M. L, Backonja, M. M, Bennett, M. I, Bouhassira, D, Cruccu, G, Hansson, P. T, et al. Assessment of neuropathic pain in primary care. Am J Med. (2009). Suppl):SEpub 2009/10/07., 13-21.

[2] Cherry, C. L, Skolasky, R. L, Lal, L, Creighton, J, Hauer, P, Raman, S. P, et al. Antiretroviral use and other risks for HIV-associated neuropathies in an international cohort. Neurology. (2006). Epub 2006/03/29., 66(6), 867-73.

[3] Murphy, R. A, Sunpath, H, Kuritzkes, D. R, Venter, F, & Gandhi, R. T. Antiretroviral therapy-associated toxicities in the resource-poor world: the challenge of a limited formulary. J Infect Dis. (2007). Suppl 3:SEpub 2008/01/10., 449-56.

[4] Croft, R. Neuropathic pain in leprosy. Int J Lepr Other Mycobact Dis. (2004). Epub 2004/08/11., 72(2), 171-2.

[5] Lacoux, P, & Ford, N. Treatment of neuropathic pain in Sierra Leone. Lancet Neurol. (2002). Epub 2003/07/10., 1(3), 190-5.

[6] Daousi, C. MacFarlane IA, Woodward A, Nurmikko TJ, Bundred PE, Benbow SJ. Chronic painful peripheral neuropathy in an urban community: a controlled comparison of people with and without diabetes. Diabet Med. (2004). Epub 2004/08/20., 21(9), 976-82.

[7] Davies, M, Brophy, S, Williams, R, & Taylor, A. The prevalence, severity, and impact of painful diabetic peripheral neuropathy in type 2 diabetes. Diabetes Care. (2006). Epub 2006/06/28., 29(7), 1518-22.

[8] Galil, K, Choo, P. W, Donahue, J. G, & Platt, R. The sequelae of herpes zoster. Arch Intern Med. (1997). Epub 1997/06/09., 157(11), 1209-13.

[9] Pachman, D. R, Barton, D. L, Watson, J. C, & Loprinzi, C. L. Chemotherapy-induced peripheral neuropathy: prevention and treatment. Clin Pharmacol Ther. (2011). Epub 2011/08/05., 90(3), 377-87.

[10] Windebank, A. J, & Grisold, W. Chemotherapy-induced neuropathy. J Peripher Nerv Syst. (2008). Epub 2008/03/19., 13(1), 27-46.

[11] Torrance, N, Smith, B. H, Bennett, M. I, & Lee, A. J. The epidemiology of chronic pain of predominantly neuropathic origin. Results from a general population survey. J Pain. (2006). Epub 2006/04/19., 7(4), 281-9.

[12] Bouhassira, D, Attal, N, Alchaar, H, Boureau, F, Brochet, B, Bruxelle, J, et al. Comparison of pain syndromes associated with nervous or somatic lesions and development of a new neuropathic pain diagnostic questionnaire (DN4). Pain. (2005). Epub 2005/03/01.

[13] Freynhagen, R, Baron, R, Gockel, U, & Tolle, T. R. painDETECT: a new screening questionnaire to identify neuropathic components in patients with back pain. Curr Med Res Opin. (2006). Epub 2006/10/07., 22(10), 1911-20.

[14] Smith, B. H, Torrance, N, Bennett, M. I, & Lee, A. J. Health and quality of life associated with chronic pain of predominantly neuropathic origin in the community. Clin J Pain. (2007). Epub 2007/01/24., 23(2), 143-9.

[15] Dworkin, R. H, Connor, O, Audette, A. B, Baron, J, Gourlay, R, & Haanpaa, G. K. ML, et al. Recommendations for the pharmacological management of neuropathic pain: an overview and literature update. Mayo Clin Proc. (2010). Suppl):SEpub 2010/03/17., 3-14.

[16] Mogil, J. S. Animal models of pain: progress and challenges. Nat Rev Neurosci. (2009). Epub 2009/03/05., 10(4), 283-94.

[17] Jensen, T. S, & Baron, R. Translation of symptoms and signs into mechanisms in neuropathic pain. Pain. (2003). Epub 2003/03/07.

[18] Treede, R. D, Jensen, T. S, Campbell, J. N, Cruccu, G, Dostrovsky, J. O, Griffin, J. W, et al. Neuropathic pain: redefinition and a grading system for clinical and research purposes. Neurology. (2008). Epub 2007/11/16., 70(18), 1630-5.

[19] Turk, D. C, Audette, J, Levy, R. M, Mackey, S. C, & Stanos, S. Assessment and treatment of psychosocial comorbidities in patients with neuropathic pain. Mayo Clin Proc. (2010). Suppl):SEpub 2010/03/17., 42-50.

[20] Baron, R. Peripheral neuropathic pain: from mechanisms to symptoms. Clin J Pain. (2000). Suppl):SEpub 2000/06/28., 12-20.

[21] Baron, R, Binder, A, & Wasner, G. Neuropathic pain: diagnosis, pathophysiological mechanisms, and treatment. Lancet Neurol. (2010). Epub 2010/07/24., 9(8), 807-19.

[22] Sherrington, C. The integrative action of the nervous system. New York: Scribner; (1906).

[23] Woolf, C. J, & Ma, Q. Nociceptors--noxious stimulus detectors. Neuron. (2007). Epub 2007/08/07., 55(3), 353-64.

[24] Caterina, M. J, Schumacher, M. A, Tominaga, M, Rosen, T. A, Levine, J. D, & Julius, D. The capsaicin receptor: a heat-activated ion channel in the pain pathway. Nature. (1997). Epub 1997/12/31 23:16., 389(6653), 816-24.

[25] Patapoutian, A, Peier, A. M, Story, G. M, & Viswanath, V. ThermoTRP channels and beyond: mechanisms of temperature sensation. Nat Rev Neurosci. (2003). Epub 2003/07/03., 4(7), 529-39.

[26] Hong, S, & Wiley, J. W. Early painful diabetic neuropathy is associated with differential changes in the expression and function of vanilloid receptor 1. J Biol Chem. (2005). Epub 2004/10/30., 280(1), 618-27.

[27] Pabbidi, R. M, Yu, S. Q, Peng, S, Khardori, R, Pauza, M. E, & Premkumar, L. S. Influence of TRPV1 on diabetes-induced alterations in thermal pain sensitivity. Mol Pain. (2008). Epub 2008/03/04.

[28] Hudson, L. J, Bevan, S, Wotherspoon, G, Gentry, C, Fox, A, & Winter, J. VR1 protein expression increases in undamaged DRG neurons after partial nerve injury. Eur J Neurosci. (2001). Epub 2001/06/26., 13(11), 2105-14.

[29] Kim, H. Y, Park, C. K, Cho, I. H, Jung, S. J, Kim, J. S, & Oh, S. B. Differential Changes in TRPV1 expression after trigeminal sensory nerve injury. J Pain. (2008). Epub 2008/01/30., 9(3), 280-8.

[30] Ta, L. E, Bieber, A. J, Carlton, S. M, Loprinzi, C. L, Low, P. A, & Windebank, A. J. Transient Receptor Potential Vanilloid 1 is essential for cisplatin-induced heat hyperalgesia in mice. Mol Pain. (2010). Epub 2010/03/09.

[31] Von Hehn, C. A, Baron, R, & Woolf, C. J. Deconstructing the neuropathic pain phenotype to reveal neural mechanisms. Neuron. (2012). Epub 2012/03/01., 73(4), 638-52.

[32] Amir, R, Michaelis, M, & Devor, M. Membrane potential oscillations in dorsal root ganglion neurons: role in normal electrogenesis and neuropathic pain. J Neurosci. (1999). Epub 1999/09/24., 19(19), 8589-96.

[33] Dib-hajj, S. D, Cummins, T. R, Black, J. A, & Waxman, S. G. Sodium channels in normal and pathological pain. Annu Rev Neurosci. (2010). Epub 2010/04/07., 33, 325-47.

[34] Krafte, D. S, & Bannon, A. W. Sodium channels and nociception: recent concepts and therapeutic opportunities. Curr Opin Pharmacol. (2008). Epub 2007/10/30., 8(1), 50-6.

[35] Rexed, B. The cytoarchitectonic organization of the spinal cord in the cat. J Comp Neurol. (1952). Epub 1952/06/01., 96(3), 414-95.

[36] Todd, A. J. Neuronal circuitry for pain processing in the dorsal horn. Nat Rev Neurosci. (2010). Epub 2010/11/12., 11(12), 823-36.

[37] Dubner, R, Hayes, R. L, & Hoffman, D. Neural and behavioral correlates of pain in the trigeminal system: In Bonica J editor: Pain, New York, (1980). Raven.

[38] Woolf, C. J. Evidence for a central component of post-injury pain hypersensitivity. Nature. (1983). Epub 1983/12/15., 306(5944), 686-8.

[39] Seal, R. P, Wang, X, Guan, Y, Raja, S. N, Woodbury, C. J, Basbaum, A. I, et al. Injury-induced mechanical hypersensitivity requires C-low threshold mechanoreceptors. Nature. (2009). Epub 2009/11/17., 462(7273), 651-5.

[40] Woolf, C. J. Central sensitization: implications for the diagnosis and treatment of pain. Pain. (2011). Suppl):SEpub 2010/10/22., 2-15.

[41] Pfau, D. B, Klein, T, Putzer, D, Pogatzki-zahn, E. M, Treede, R. D, & Magerl, W. Analysis of hyperalgesia time courses in humans after painful electrical high-frequency stimulation identifies a possible transition from early to late LTP-like pain plasticity. Pain. (2011). Epub 2011/03/29., 152(7), 1532-9.

[42] Ji, R. R, Kohno, T, Moore, K. A, & Woolf, C. J. Central sensitization and LTP: do pain and memory share similar mechanisms? Trends Neurosci. (2003). Epub 2003/11/20., 26(12), 696-705.

[43] Nitzan-luques, A, Devor, M, & Tal, M. Genotype-selective phenotypic switch in primary afferent neurons contributes to neuropathic pain. Pain. (2011). Epub 2011/08/30., 152(10), 2413-26.

[44] Tan, A. M, Chang, Y. W, Zhao, P, Hains, B. C, & Waxman, S. G. Rac1-regulated dendritic spine remodeling contributes to neuropathic pain after peripheral nerve injury. Exp Neurol. (2011). Epub 2011/10/04., 232(2), 222-33.

[45] Baba, H, Ji, R. R, Kohno, T, Moore, K. A, Ataka, T, Wakai, A, et al. Removal of GABAergic inhibition facilitates polysynaptic A fiber-mediated excitatory transmission to the superficial spinal dorsal horn. Mol Cell Neurosci. (2003). Epub 2003/12/11., 24(3), 818-30.

[46] Scholz, J, Broom, D. C, Youn, D. H, Mills, C. D, Kohno, T, Suter, M. R, et al. Blocking caspase activity prevents transsynaptic neuronal apoptosis and the loss of inhibition in lamina II of the dorsal horn after peripheral nerve injury. J Neurosci. (2005). Epub 2005/08/12., 25(32), 7317-23.

[47] De Felice, M, Sanoja, R, Wang, R, Vera-portocarrero, L, Oyarzo, J, King, T, et al. Engagement of descending inhibition from the rostral ventromedial medulla protects against chronic neuropathic pain. Pain. (2011). Epub 2011/07/13., 152(12), 2701-9.

[48] Polgar, E, Gray, S, Riddell, J. S, & Todd, A. J. Lack of evidence for significant neuronal loss in laminae I-III of the spinal dorsal horn of the rat in the chronic constriction injury model. Pain. (2004). Epub 2004/08/26.

[49] Polgar, E, Hughes, D. I, Arham, A. Z, & Todd, A. J. Loss of neurons from laminas I-III of the spinal dorsal horn is not required for development of tactile allodynia in the spared nerve injury model of neuropathic pain. J Neurosci. (2005). Epub 2005/07/15., 25(28), 6658-66.

[50] Polgar, E, Hughes, D. I, Riddell, J. S, Maxwell, D. J, Puskar, Z, & Todd, A. J. Selective loss of spinal GABAergic or glycinergic neurons is not necessary for development of thermal hyperalgesia in the chronic constriction injury model of neuropathic pain. Pain. (2003). Epub 2003/07/12.

[51] Watkins, L. R, Milligan, E. D, & Maier, S. F. Glial activation: a driving force for pathological pain. Trends Neurosci. (2001). Epub 2001/07/31., 24(8), 450-5.

[52] Coull, J. A, Beggs, S, Boudreau, D, Boivin, D, Tsuda, M, Inoue, K, et al. BDNF from microglia causes the shift in neuronal anion gradient underlying neuropathic pain. Nature. (2005). Epub 2005/12/16., 438(7070), 1017-21.

[53] Apkarian, A. V, Hashmi, J. A, & Baliki, M. N. Pain and the brain: specificity and plasticity of the brain in clinical chronic pain. Pain. (2011). Suppl):SEpub 2010/12/15., 49-64.

[54] Rainville, P, Duncan, G. H, Price, D. D, Carrier, B, & Bushnell, M. C. Pain affect encoded in human anterior cingulate but not somatosensory cortex. Science. (1997). Epub 1997/08/15., 277(5328), 968-71.

[55] Hofbauer, R. K, Rainville, P, Duncan, G. H, & Bushnell, M. C. Cortical representation of the sensory dimension of pain. J Neurophysiol. (2001). Epub 2001/06/30., 86(1), 402-11.

[56] Baliki, M. N, Geha, P. Y, & Apkarian, A. V. Parsing pain perception between nociceptive representation and magnitude estimation. J Neurophysiol. (2009). Epub 2008/12/17., 101(2), 875-87.

[57] Apkarian, A. V, Sosa, Y, Sonty, S, Levy, R. M, Harden, R. N, Parrish, T. B, et al. Chronic back pain is associated with decreased prefrontal and thalamic gray matter density. J Neurosci. (2004). Epub 2004/11/19., 24(46), 10410-5.

[58] Davis, K. D, Pope, G, Chen, J, Kwan, C. L, Crawley, A. P, & Diamant, N. E. Cortical thinning in IBS: implications for homeostatic, attention, and pain processing. Neurology. (2008). Epub 2007/10/26., 70(2), 153-4.

[59] Hsu, M. C, Harris, R. E, Sundgren, P. C, Welsh, R. C, Fernandes, C. R, Clauw, D. J, et al. No consistent difference in gray matter volume between individuals with fibromyalgia and age-matched healthy subjects when controlling for affective disorder. Pain. (2009). Epub 2009/04/21., 143(3), 262-7.

[60] Kuchinad, A, Schweinhardt, P, Seminowicz, D. A, Wood, P. B, Chizh, B. A, & Bushnell, M. C. Accelerated brain gray matter loss in fibromyalgia patients: premature aging of the brain? J Neurosci. (2007). Epub 2007/04/13., 27(15), 4004-7.

[61] Luerding, R, Weigand, T, Bogdahn, U, & Schmidt-wilcke, T. Working memory performance is correlated with local brain morphology in the medial frontal and anterior cingulate cortex in fibromyalgia patients: structural correlates of pain-cognition interaction. Brain. (2008). Pt 12):3222-31. Epub 2008/09/30.

[62] Schmidt-wilcke, T, Leinisch, E, Straube, A, Kampfe, N, Draganski, B, Diener, H. C, et al. Gray matter decrease in patients with chronic tension type headache. Neurology. (2005). Epub 2005/11/09., 65(9), 1483-6.

[63] Rodriguez-raecke, R, Niemeier, A, Ihle, K, Ruether, W, & May, A. Brain gray matter decrease in chronic pain is the consequence and not the cause of pain. J Neurosci. (2009). Epub 2009/11/06., 29(44), 13746-50.

[64] Suzuki, M, Nohara, S, Hagino, H, Kurokawa, K, Yotsutsuji, T, Kawasaki, Y, et al. Regional changes in brain gray and white matter in patients with schizophrenia demonstrated with voxel-based analysis of MRI. Schizophr Res. (2002). Epub 2002/04/17.

[65] Schmidt-wilcke, T, Luerding, R, Weigand, T, Jurgens, T, Schuierer, G, Leinisch, E, et al. Striatal grey matter increase in patients suffering from fibromyalgia--a voxel-based morphometry study. Pain. (2007). Suppl 1:SEpub 2007/06/26., 109-16.

[66] Valfre, W, Rainero, I, Bergui, M, & Pinessi, L. Voxel-based morphometry reveals gray matter abnormalities in migraine. Headache. (2008). Epub 2008/01/11., 48(1), 109-17.

[67] Gwilym, S. E, Filippini, N, Douaud, G, Carr, A. J, & Tracey, I. Thalamic atrophy associated with painful osteoarthritis of the hip is reversible after arthroplasty: a longitudinal voxel-based morphometric study. Arthritis Rheum. (2010). Epub 2010/06/03., 62(10), 2930-40.

[68] Obermann, M, Nebel, K, Schumann, C, Holle, D, Gizewski, E. R, Maschke, M, et al. Gray matter changes related to chronic posttraumatic headache. Neurology. (2009). Epub 2009/09/23., 73(12), 978-83.

[69] Baliki, M. N, Geha, P. Y, Apkarian, A. V, & Chialvo, D. R. Beyond feeling: chronic pain hurts the brain, disrupting the default-mode network dynamics. J Neurosci. (2008). Epub 2008/02/08., 28(6), 1398-403.

[70] Mantyselka, P, Kumpusalo, E, Ahonen, R, Kumpusalo, A, Kauhanen, J, Viinamaki, H, et al. Pain as a reason to visit the doctor: a study in Finnish primary health care. Pain. (2001). Epub 2001/02/13.

[71] Connor, O. AB. Neuropathic pain: quality-of-life impact, costs and cost effectiveness of therapy. Pharmacoeconomics. (2009). Epub 2009/03/04., 27(2), 95-112.

[72] Berger, A, Dukes, E. M, & Oster, G. Clinical characteristics and economic costs of patients with painful neuropathic disorders. J Pain. (2004). Epub 2004/04/24., 5(3), 143-9.

[73] Dworkin, R. H, White, R, Connor, O, Baser, A. B, & Hawkins, O. K. Healthcare costs of acute and chronic pain associated with a diagnosis of herpes zoster. J Am Geriatr Soc. (2007). Epub 2007/07/31., 55(8), 1168-75.

[74] Dworkin, R. H, Malone, D. C, Panarites, C. J, Armstrong, E. P, & Pham, S. V. Impact of postherpetic neuralgia and painful diabetic peripheral neuropathy on health care costs. J Pain. (2010). Epub 2009/10/27., 11(4), 360-8.

[75] Woolf, C. J, & Mannion, R. J. Neuropathic pain: aetiology, symptoms, mechanisms, and management. Lancet. 1999;Epub (1999). , 353(9168), 1959-64.

[76] Finnerup, N. B, & Jensen, T. S. Mechanisms of disease: mechanism-based classification of neuropathic pain-a critical analysis. Nat Clin Pract Neurol. (2006). Epub 2006/08/26., 2(2), 107-15.

[77] Woolf, C. J. Dissecting out mechanisms responsible for peripheral neuropathic pain: implications for diagnosis and therapy. Life Sci. (2004). Epub 2004/03/26., 74(21), 2605-10.

[78] Stacey, B. R, Barrett, J. A, Whalen, E, Phillips, K. F, & Rowbotham, M. C. Pregabalin for postherpetic neuralgia: placebo-controlled trial of fixed and flexible dosing regimens on allodynia and time to onset of pain relief. J Pain. (2008). Epub 2008/07/22., 9(11), 1006-17.

[79] Bennett, M. The LANSS Pain Scale: the Leeds assessment of neuropathic symptoms and signs. Pain. (2001). Epub 2001/04/27.

[80] Bennett, M. I, Attal, N, Backonja, M. M, Baron, R, Bouhassira, D, Freynhagen, R, et al. Using screening tools to identify neuropathic pain. Pain. (2007). Epub 2006/12/22., 127(3), 199-203.

[81] Dworkin, R. H, Connor, O, Backonja, A. B, Farrar, M, Finnerup, J. T, & Jensen, N. B. TS, et al. Pharmacologic management of neuropathic pain: evidence-based recommendations. Pain. (2007). Epub 2007/10/09., 132(3), 237-51.

[82] Finnerup, N. B, Otto, M, Mcquay, H. J, Jensen, T. S, & Sindrup, S. H. Algorithm for neuropathic pain treatment: an evidence based proposal. Pain. (2005). Epub 2005/10/11., 118(3), 289-305.

[83] Maneuf, Y. P, Luo, Z. D, & Lee, K. alpha2delta and the mechanism of action of gabapentin in the treatment of pain. Semin Cell Dev Biol. (2006). Epub 2006/10/28., 17(5), 565-70.

[84] Wu, C. L, Agarwal, S, Tella, P. K, Klick, B, Clark, M. R, Haythornthwaite, J. A, et al. Morphine versus mexiletine for treatment of postamputation pain: a randomized,

placebo-controlled, crossover trial. Anesthesiology. (2008). Epub 2008/07/24., 109(2), 289-96.

[85] Tugnoli, V, Capone, J. G, Eleopra, R, Quatrale, R, Sensi, M, Gastaldo, E, et al. Botulinum toxin type A reduces capsaicin-evoked pain and neurogenic vasodilatation in human skin. Pain. (2007). Epub 2006/12/30.

[86] Ranoux, D, Attal, N, Morain, F, & Bouhassira, D. Botulinum toxin type A induces direct analgesic effects in chronic neuropathic pain. Ann Neurol. (2008). Epub 2008/06/12., 64(3), 274-83.

[87] Rauck, R. L, Shaibani, A, Biton, V, Simpson, J, & Koch, B. Lacosamide in painful diabetic peripheral neuropathy: a phase 2 double-blind placebo-controlled study. Clin J Pain. (2007). Epub 2007/01/24., 23(2), 150-8.

[88] Shaibani, A, Fares, S, Selam, J. L, Arslanian, A, Simpson, J, Sen, D, et al. Lacosamide in painful diabetic neuropathy: an 18-week double-blind placebo-controlled trial. J Pain. (2009). Epub 2009/05/05., 10(8), 818-28.

[89] Wymer, J. P, Simpson, J, Sen, D, & Bongardt, S. Efficacy and safety of lacosamide in diabetic neuropathic pain: an 18-week double-blind placebo-controlled trial of fixed-dose regimens. Clin J Pain. (2009). Epub 2009/05/21., 25(5), 376-85.

[90] Dhanani, N. M, Caruso, T. J, & Carinci, A. J. Complementary and alternative medicine for pain: an evidence-based review. Curr Pain Headache Rep. (2011). Epub 2010/11/11., 15(1), 39-46.

[91] Bittar, R. G, Kar-purkayastha, I, Owen, S. L, Bear, R. E, Green, A, Wang, S, et al. Deep brain stimulation for pain relief: a meta-analysis. J Clin Neurosci. (2005). Epub 2005/07/05., 12(5), 515-9.

[92] Mallory, G. W, Huang, S. C, Gorman, D. A, Stead, S. M, Klassen, B. T, Watson, J. C, & Lee, K. H. The nucleus accumbens as a potential target for central post-stroke pain. Mayo Clinic Proceedings. (In Press).

[93] Marineo, G, Iorno, V, Gandini, C, Moschini, V, & Smith, T. J. Scrambler therapy may relieve chronic neuropathic pain more effectively than guideline-based drug management: results of a pilot, randomized, controlled trial. J Pain Symptom Manage. (2012). Epub 2011/07/19., 43(1), 87-95.

[94] Smith, T. J, Coyne, P. J, Parker, G. L, Dodson, P, & Ramakrishnan, V. Pilot trial of a patient-specific cutaneous electrostimulation device (MC5-A Calmare(R)) for chemotherapy-induced peripheral neuropathy. J Pain Symptom Manage. (2010). Epub 2010/09/04., 40(6), 883-91.

[95] Rehm, S. E, Koroschetz, J, Gockel, U, Brosz, M, Freynhagen, R, Tolle, T. R, et al. A cross-sectional survey of 3035 patients with fibromyalgia: subgroups of patients with typical comorbidities and sensory symptom profiles. Rheumatology (Oxford). (2010). Epub 2010/03/20., 49(6), 1146-52.

[96] Costigan, M, Scholz, J, & Woolf, C. J. Neuropathic pain: a maladaptive response of the nervous system to damage. Annu Rev Neurosci. (2009). Epub 2009/04/30., 32, 1-32.

[97] Diatchenko, L, Slade, G. D, Nackley, A. G, Bhalang, K, Sigurdsson, A, Belfer, I, et al. Genetic basis for individual variations in pain perception and the development of a chronic pain condition. Hum Mol Genet. (2005). Epub 2004/11/13., 14(1), 135-43.

[98] Nackley, A. G, Shabalina, S. A, Tchivileva, I. E, Satterfield, K, Korchynskyi, O, Makarov, S. S, et al. Human catechol-O-methyltransferase haplotypes modulate protein expression by altering mRNA secondary structure. Science. (2006). Epub 2006/12/23., 314(5807), 1930-3.

[99] Lotsch, J, & Geisslinger, G. Current evidence for a modulation of nociception by human genetic polymorphisms. Pain. (2007). Epub 2007/08/21.

[100] Mogil, J. S, Wilson, S. G, Chesler, E. J, Rankin, A. L, Nemmani, K. V, Lariviere, W. R, et al. The melanocortin-1 receptor gene mediates female-specific mechanisms of analgesia in mice and humans. Proc Natl Acad Sci U S A. (2003). Epub 2003/03/29., 100(8), 4867-72.

[101] Tegeder, I, Costigan, M, Griffin, R. S, Abele, A, Belfer, I, Schmidt, H, et al. GTP cyclohydrolase and tetrahydrobiopterin regulate pain sensitivity and persistence. Nat Med. (2006). Epub 2006/10/24., 12(11), 1269-77.

Chapter 2

From Animal Models to Clinical Practicality: Lessons Learned from Current Translational Progress of Diabetic Peripheral Neuropathy

Chengyuan Li, Anne E. Bunner and John J. Pippin

Additional information is available at the end of the chapter

http://dx.doi.org/10.5772/55364

1. Introduction

1.1. Overview of DPN

In diabetes mellitus, nerves and their supporting cells are subjected to prolonged hyperglycemia and metabolic disturbances and this culminates in reversible/irreversible nervous system dysfunction and damage, namely diabetic peripheral neuropathy (DPN). Due to the varying compositions and extents of neurological involvements, it is difficult to obtain accurate and thorough prevalence estimates of DPN, rendering this microvascular complication vastly underdiagnosed and undertreated [1-4]. According to American Diabetes Association, DPN occurs to 60-70% of diabetic individuals [5] and represents the leading cause of peripheral neuropathies among all cases [6, 7]. As the incidence of diabetes is approaching global epidemic level, its neurological consequences are estimated to affect some $300 million people worldwide [8] and costs 15 billion dollars on annual health-care expenditures in the U.S. alone [9].

1.1.1. A Complex natural history

Because diverse anatomic distributions and fiber types may be differentially affected in patients with diabetes, the disease manifestations, courses and pathologies of clinical and subclinical DPN are rather heterogeneous and encompass a broad spectrum [1, 10, 11]. Additionally, dietary influences, risk covariates, genetic and phenotypic multiplicity further perplex the definition, diagnosis, classification and natural history of DPN [6, 10, 12, 13]. Current consensus divides diabetes-associated somatic neuropathic syndromes into the focal/multifocal and diffuse/generalized neuropathies [6, 14]. The first category comprises a group of asymmetrical, acute-in-onset and self-limited single lesion(s) of nerve injury or impairment largely resulting from the increased vulnerability of diabetic nerves to mechanical insults (Carpal Tunnel Syndrome) (reviewed in 15). Such mononeuropathies occur idiopathically and only become a clinical problem in association with aging in 5-10% of those affected. Therefore, focal neuropathies are not extensively covered in this chapter [16]. The rest of the patients frequently develop diffuse neuropathies characterized by symmetrical distribution, insidious onset and chronic progression. In particular, a distal symmetrical sensorimotor polyneuropathy accounts for 90% of all DPN diagnoses in type 1 and type 2 diabetics and affects all types of peripheral sensory and motor fibers in a temporally non-uniform manner [6, 17].

Symptoms begin with prickling, tingling, numbness, paresthesia, dysesthesia and various qualities of pain associated with small sensory fibers at the very distal end (toes) of lower extremities [1, 18]. Presence of the above symptoms together with abnormal nociceptive response of epidermal C and A-δ fibers to pain/temperature (as revealed by clinical examination) constitute the diagnosis of small fiber sensory neuropathy, which produces both painful and insensate phenotypes [19]. Painful diabetic neuropathy is a prominent, distressing and chronic experience in at least 10-30% of DPN populations [20, 21]. Its occurrence does not necessarily correlate with impairment in electrophysiological or quantitative sensory testing (QST). Some have suggested pain to reflect the pathobiological changes of serum glucose level at least in individuals with pre- or recent diagnosis. Consistent with this notion, severe neuropathic pain often presents as a typical feature in acute reversible sensory/hyperglycemic neuropathy and its onset and remission following glycemic control can be indicative of spontaneous repair of nerve damage in the early phase of DPN [1, 10, 22, 23]. Pain in many diabetics may persist, however, only to be alleviated as progressive and irreversible nerve deterioration and loss of thermal sensitivity take place [10, 21]. Large myelinated sensory fibers that innervate the dermis, such as Aβ, also become involved later on, leading to impaired proprioception, vibration and tactile detection, and mechanical hypoalgesia [19]. Following this "stocking-glove", length-dependent and dying-back evolvement, neurodegeneration gradually proceeds to proximal muscle sensory and motor nerves. Its presence manifests in neurological testings as reduced nerve impulse conductions, diminished ankle tendon reflex, unsteadiness and muscle weakness [1, 24].

Both the absence of protective sensory response and motor coordination predispose neuropathic foot to impaired wound healing and gangrenous ulceration—often ensued by limb amputation in severe and/or advanced cases [25, 26]. This traumatic procedure is performed on approximately 100,000 Americans every year and is a major attributing factor for diabetes-related hospital bed occupancy and medical expenses [27]. Although symptomatic motor deficits only appear in later stages of DPN [25], motor denervation and distal atrophy can increase the rate of fractures by causing repetitive minor trauma or falls [24, 28]. Other unusual but highly disabling late sequelae of DPN include limb ischemia and joint deformity [6]; the latter also being termed Charcot's neuroarthropathy or Charcot's joints [1]. In addition to significant morbidities, several separate cohort studies provided evidence that DPN [29], diabetic foot ulcers [30] and increased toe vibration perception threshold (VPT) [31] are all independent risk factors for mortality. Overall, neuropathic pain, foot complication as well as various associated psychosocial comorbidities inflict a significant diminution on the quality and duration of life of individuals affected by DPN, which in turn is raising an escalating health, social and economic problem in both developed and developing countries [4, 14].

1.2. A medical challenge

Unfortunately, current therapy for DPN is far from effective and at best only delays the onset and/or progression of the disease via tight glucose control, the only established means for managing diabetic complications in the U.S. Several large-scale, multicenter and landmark clinical studies, including Diabetes Control and Complication Trial, provided irrefutable evidence that chronic hyperglycemia is a leading factor in the etiology and treatment of DPN [32-36]. However, euglycemia cannot always be achieved through aggressive insulin therapy or other anti-diabetic agents. Even with near normoglycemic control, a substantial proportion of patients still suffer the debilitating neurotoxic consequences of diabetes [34]. On the other hand, some with poor glucose control are spared from clinically evident signs and symptoms of neuropathy for a long time after diagnosis [37-39]. Thus, other etiological factors independent of hyperglycemia are likely to be involved in the development of DPN. Data from a number of prospective, observational studies suggested that older age, longer diabetes duration, genetic polymorphism, presence of cardiovascular disease markers, malnutrition, presence of other microvascular complications, alcohol and tobacco consumption, and higher constitutional indexes (e.g. weight and height) interact with diabetes and make for strong predictors of neurological decline [13, 32, 40-42]. Targeting some of these modifiable risk factors in addition to glycemia may improve the management of DPN.

Meanwhile, enormous efforts have been devoted to understanding and intervening with the molecular and biochemical processes linking the metabolic disturbances to sensorimotor deficits by studying diabetic animal models. In return, nearly 2,200 articles were published in PubMed central and at least 100 clinical trials were reported evaluating the efficacy of a number of pharmacological agents; the majority of them are designed to inhibit specific pathogenic mechanisms identified by these experimental approaches. Candidate agents have included aldose reductase inhibitors, AGE inhibitors, γ-linolenic acid, α-lipoic acid, vasodilators, nerve growth factor, protein kinase Cβ inhibitors, and vascular endothelial growth factor. Notwithstanding a fruitful of knowledge and promising results in animals, none has translated into definitive clinical success (Figure 1). While the notorious biochemical heterogeneity and temporal non-uniformity of the disease processes among and even within individuals can take much of the blame, investigators must take into serious consideration the marked differences between animals and humans, which may substantially impair the application of experimental data to clinical settings. The following sections of this chapter describe the clinical outcomes of these pathogenetic treatments that put previous observations generated by animal studies into perspective, and discuss the molecular, cellular and physiological roots underlying the limited translation.

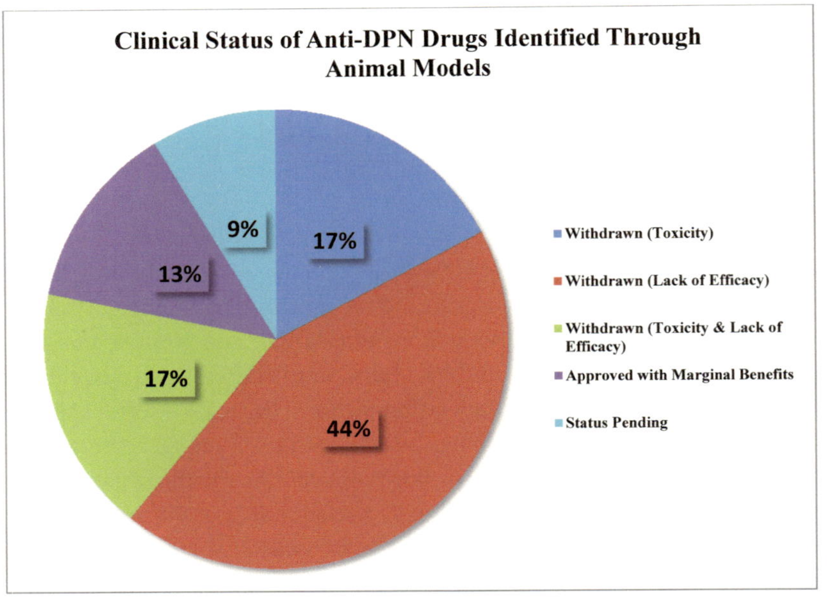

Figure 1. Summary of Current Clinical Status of Anti-DPN Drugs Developed via Animal Models. Data are generated from published experimental and clinical results to date on pharmacological agents (a total of 23 drugs) targeting pathogenetic mechanisms listed in but not limited to section 2.

2. Pharmacological management of DPN via targeting pathogenetic mechanisms: From animal models to clinical practice

2.1. Managing metabolic derangements

2.1.1. Polyol pathway and aldose reductase inhibitors

Polyol pathway arose as a plausible link of glucose dismetabolism to DPN in middle 1960s [43] and has received much interest due to the strong evidence accumulating from experimental diabetic rats [44]. Two consecutive oxidoreductive reactions essentially constitute the polyol pathway: the rate-limiting NADPH-dependent aldose reductase (AR) reduces glucose to sorbitol, which then becomes the substrate for NAD^+-dependent sorbitol dehydrogenase (SDH) and oxidized into fructose. Although AR has a high K_M for glucose under the physiological condition, hyperglysolia (high intracellular glucose concentration) can excessively activate this enzyme resulting in a nearly 4-fold induction in glucose disposal through this pathway in human erythrocytes [45, 46]. Because these polyhydroxylated alcohols have little transmembrane diffusibility, their retention within ocular lens fibrils of hyperglycemic rats or rabbits was proposed to cause hyperosmotic perturbation of intracellular metabolites, electrolytes and other osmolytes and subsequent hydropic cataractogenesis as observed. All

http://dx.doi.org/10.5772/55364

of these were preventable and reversible by blocking AR [47-51]. In mice, transgenic overexpression of the gene encoding human AR (hAR) in lens epithelia submitted these cataract-resistant animals to sugar-induced polyol deposit and cataract formation, which became more acute when coupled with genetic SDH deficiency [52]. Studies of type 1 and type 2 diabetes models, including alloxan- and streptozotocin (STZ)-induced diabetic rats and leptin-deficient *ob/ob* mice, soon confirmed a significant elevation of sorbitol and fructose in sciatic nerves, dorsal root ganglia (DRGs) and spinal cord. This correlated with nerve/axonal conduction and transport deficiencies, loss of intraepidermal nerve fibers, increased neural and endoneurial oxidative-nitrosative stress as well as thermal hypoalgesia and tactile allodynia [43, 53-57]. A "polyol hypothesis" derived from diabetic lens was thus propelled to the pathogenesis of DPN [47]. In keeping with this notion, AR inhibitors that reduce nerve polyol levels showed remarkable preservation of nerve structure and function in rats with either spontaneous or chemical-induced diabetes [53, 58-60]. Systemic hAR overexpression combined with STZ-induced diabetes led to an exacerbated but AR inhibitor-preventable peripheral nerve sorbitol and fructose buildup, electroactivity suppression and myelinated fiber atrophy [61]. A similar biochemical and electrophysiological but not morphological abnormality was obtained with Schwann cell (SC)-targeted hAR transgenic mice, indicating that SC AR hyperactivity contributes to many, though not all pathological change of DPN [62]. Conversely, AR-knockout mice showed no obvious sorbitol accumulation, conduction slowing, oxidative stress, or stress kinase activation. Additionally, there were fewer loss of sural nerve fibers in AR-deficient mice compared to wild-types (WTs) [63]. Since galactose has approximately 4 times higher affinity for AR than glucose [64] and its reduction product galactitol is poorly disposed, galactose-rich diet was used as a popular substitute for classical hyperglycemic models to exemplify and examine the role of excessive polyalcohol formation in the genesis of diabetic cataract and neuropathy [47]. Along the line with "aldo-osmotic theory", galactosemic rodents that accrue much greater level of this alternate AR metabolite also exhibit similar and sometimes more severe electrophysiological, anatomical and biochemical defects that are seen diabetic models [65-67]. However, galactosemia is a rare metabolic condition in humans (less than 0.002% of the population) [68] and the galactosemic lens and nerves often manifest functional and structural lesions resulting from acute and exaggerated galactitol intoxication that differ from those of diabetic cataract and neuropathy [47, 69-71]. Hence, galactose-fed animals are neither appropriate models for studying diabetic complications nor good replacements for characterizing the pathogenetic involvement of sorbitol pathway in these conditions. Other studies further revealed that neither the morphometrical [59] nor functional indices in DPN correlate with the tissue sorbitol content [72, 73]. Instead, nerve myo-inositol content is more closely related to the neurophysiological function according to most reports. Depletion of cytoplasmic myo-inositol, protein kinase C activation and tubulin/Na^+/K^+-ATPase complex formation were proposed mechanisms that mediate polyol pathway overflow-induced impairment of Na^+/K^+-ATPase ion pumping and subsequent reduction of nerve conduction velocity (NCV) [45, 55, 74]. In addition, augmented cofactor consumption by AR and SDH not only deprives glutathione reductase of NADPH and the capacity to regenerate reduced glutathione (GSH) [45] but also contributes to an imbalanced redox state of NADH/NAD^+ [75], thus promoting oxidative and vascular injury [63, 76, 77].

Overall, the above and numerous other observations obtained from the use of animal models demonstrated consistently that increased polyol metabolism is a strong and readily reversible component in the pathogenesis of diabetes-induced degenerative changes. However, data from human studies indicated no convincing association between the elevation of glucose flux via AR and neuropathic development. Whereas nerves from amputated limbs of diabetic individuals contained significantly higher concentrations of sorbitol and fructose than non-diabetics [78], an assessment of sural nerve biopsies by Dyck *et al.* found that over two thirds of subjects with mild to severe clinical signs or symptoms of DPN had a normal polyol content [79]. A later study by the same group was able to show an inverse relationship between nerve sorbitol level and myelinated fiber density but not other neurological parameters [80]. Importantly, none of the nerve specimen analyses identified a decrease in myo-inositols in relation to DPN, in contrast with the invariable observations of myo-inositol deficiency in rodent models. Likewise, dietary supplementation of myo-inositol prevented and reversed a variety of pathophysiological processes associated with early DPN in rats [81, 82] but failed to normalize any peripheral nerve deterioration in patients with a recent diabetes onset [83, 84]. Nevertheless, the prominent success of AR inhibitors (ARIs) in preventing and reversing experimental diabetic cataract and neuropathy [58, 60, 85-89] as well as the findings of AR gene polymorphisms in diabetic microvascular complication [90-93] spurred a broad enthusiasm in the clinical exploration of these ARIs. While the use of various ARIs almost always prevented or reversed the lens opacification in diabetic rats [94], whether they can reduce the risk of cataract formation in human diabetics remains unclear. This is because most experimentally induced diabetic cataracts occur acutely and possess distinct morphological alterations similar to the features seen with the rare juvenile form of diabetic cataract. Contrasting the juvenile form, the majority of cataracts in diabetes has a dubious sorbitol increase and is represented by the slow, refractive cataract change in diabetic adults [95]. Therefore, a direct evaluation of the use of ARIs as an anti-cataract treatment is difficult in these animal models.

With regard to DPN, two earliest ARIs to be tested for their clinical efficacy in treating DPN were Alrestatin and Sorbinil, which were the prototypic ARIs belonging to the chemical classes of succinimide and spirohydantoins, respectively. Alrestatin produced minor subjective benefit but no improvement on NCV or other objective examinations [96, 97]. While Sorbinil moderately reduced the NCV decline and increased the density of regenerating myelinated fibers in sural nerves [98, 99], its influence on pain and vagal function is questionable and no meaningful therapeutic effects were experienced by patients with diabetic autonomic or polyneuropathy [100-102]. Both Sorbinil and Alrestatin were withdrawn from the clinical setting due to a high rate of toxicity involving photosensitive skin rash [1, 14]. Tolrestat, an acetic acid compound, was able to halt the progression of subclinical peripheral and autonomic deficits in a 52-week duration but had only a mild benefit on chronic symptomatic sensori-motor neuropathy [103-106]. The poor electrophysiological outcome and the incidence of fatal hepatic necrosis eventually led to discontinuation of Tolrestat study [107]. In the cases of the carboxylic acid class of ARIs, Ponalrestat manifested minimal tissue penetration and nerve sorbitol reduction, in spite of its good pharmacokinetics and pharmacodynamics in diabetic rats [108-110]. Although Zopolrestat and Zenarestat demonstrated a dose-dependent amelio-ration in NCV deficits, both of them failed to significantly improve the clinical endpoints without causing serious adverse reactions [111, 112]. Ranirestat, or As-3201, emerged as a spirosuccinimide with a better drug profile, and was effective in increasing NCVs and sensory function in a phase II trial of mild to moderate diabetic sensorimotor polyneuropathy [113]. The large-scale long-term Phase III trial of Ranirestat, however, did not show statistically significant differences in sensory parameters compared to placebo at all doses tested [114]. Another spirohydantoin, Fidarestat, displayed increased tolerability and a similar degree of improvement in subjective measures to that of Sorbinil [115]. After phase III evaluation, a minor therapeutic value was concluded for Fidarestat in the literatures and its further development was suspended for financial reasons [14, 116]. To date, Epalrestat is the only ARI approved for clinical use in Japan. Despite its success in delaying nerve conduction and sensory abnormalities in a randomized, open label, controlled multicenter trial among Japanese patients [117], the efficacy of Epalrestat has not been confirmed in other populations and appears only marginal in other documentations [1, 118]. In an attempt to identify a meaningful treatment effect of ARIs for clinical DPN, Chalk *et al* conducted a meta-analysis for 13 trials of ARIs involving 879 treated participants and 909 controls. This report found no difference in the overall outcome (SMD -0.25, 95% CI -0.56 to 0.05), nerve conduction parameters or foot ulcers between treatment and control group [119]. Similarly, a previous meta-analysis of studies published before 1996 testing four different ARIs indicated that AR inhibition achieved less than 1 m/s offsets in the decline of median and peroneal motor nerve conduction velocity (MNCV) as the single true statistical change [120]. Given these inconclusive results and safety issues, FDA has not approved any of the aforementioned agents for pharmacological intervention of DPN. Although a number of confounding factors, including unexpected placebo effect and trial design, have been blamed for the disappointing clinical outcome, the lack of clear sensory protection by ARIs puts the relevance of polyol pathway to DPN into question.

2.1.2. *Advanced glycation and aminoguanidine*

Animal and cell studies have well established the contribution of advanced glycation end products (AGEs) to diabetic tissue damage. Nerves, retina and kidney do not depend on insulin for glucose uptake and absorb this energy substrate as a direct function of the circulating glucose concentration. Prolonged hyperglysolia cultivates the glucose autoxidation, decomposition of the Amadori products (fructosamines) following adduction of glucose to the amino groups of lysine residues in the proteins, and fragmentation of glycolytic intermediates (such as glyceraldehyde-3-phosphate and dihydroxyacetone phosphate). All of these gives rise to glyoxal, 3-deoxyglucosone and methylglyoxal within the cells [121]. These highly reducing dicarbonyls are AGE precursors or glycating agents that non-enzymatically react with intracellular nucleotides, proteins, lipids, extracellular matrix and plasma components [122]. The last one is best reflected by the elevated serum glycosylated hemoglobin [HbA1c] level in diabetes. AGE modification of growth factors [123], endocytotic proteins [124], cytoskeletal actin and filaments [125, 126], interstitial matrix and adhesive molecules [127] as well as serum albumin [128] were found in increased amounts in hyperglycemia-treated endothelial cells or diabetic rats and these associated with increased vascular damage, endocytosis, cytoskeletal disassembly, fluid filtration and albuminuria. In both human diabetics and STZ-rats, there was enhanced AGE deposition in peripheral nerves compared to healthy controls as indicated by immunohistochemical assay [129, 130]. Particularly, pentosidine, a long-lived AGE marker, was significantly elevated in the cytoskeletal protein extracts isolated from diabetic subjects [130, 131]. Moreover, nerve specimens that harvest more AGEs also manifest lower myelinated fiber density.

With respect to intervention, aminoguanidine was the earliest chemical characterized for its anti-glycation activity. It is a hydrazine that preferably and competitively binds to AGE precursors and prevents further irreversible protein glycation [132]. Later studies discovered that besides inhibition of AGE formation, aminoguanidine can negatively act on inducible nitric oxide synthase [133], amine oxidase [134] and reactive oxygen species [135]. Such plethoric pharmacological properties suggest that aminoguanidine is not an appropriate investigational tool for the role of advance glycation in diabetic pathology. However, the continuous use of this compound in preclinical and clinical research was justified by its promising therapeutic effects in rat model of diabetic nephropathy [136], retinopathy [136] and neuropathy [137]. Whereas treating diabetic rats with various doses of aminoguanidine prevented or ameliorated the decrease in nerve blood flow, slowing of NCVs, endoneurial microvessel expansion and failure of sensory nerve regeneration [137-141], subcutaneous injection of aminoguanidine did not improve any of the structural or functional abnormalities in STZ-induced type I diabetic baboons [142]. Although the authors concluded that accumulation of AGEs is not likely an early mechanism of nerve damage in DPN, this discrepancy may also reflect considerable species differences. Indeed, none of the large standardized clinical trials proved a significant advantage of aminoguanidine over placebo in patients, who had well-established diabetic nephropathy [143, 144]. Rather, aminoguanidine adversely affected gastrointestinal, hepatic, respiratory and immune functions and finally led to termination of the studies. For these reasons, no further evaluation of the efficacy of aminoguanidine in treating DPN was pursued.

2.2. Blocking signaling conducers

2.2.1. Protein kinase C and ruboxistaurin

Protein kinase C (PKC) is a ubiquitous serine/threonine kinase of numerous isoforms and cellular functions. Observations in retinal and glomerular tissues from diabetic animals *in vitro* and *in vivo* support the hypothesis that elevated glycolysis subsequent to hyperglycemia dramatically raises 1,2-diacylglycerol (DAG) synthesis. In turn, DAG activates a majority of PKC family members, including PKC-α and -β [45]. Enhanced expression and activity of PKC isoforms, primarily PKC-β, pathologically affect vascular contractility and permeability thereby compromising microcirculation and causing microvascular occlusion [14, 145]. These deleterious consequences have been suggested by many to contribute to the vascular insults and development of retinopathy, nephropathy and cardiovascular disorder in diabetes. However, DAG and PKC upregulation is not a uniform pattern of change in every complication-prone tissue. Unlike the findings in nonneural diabetic complications, nerve DAG levels fall in diabetes and experimental rodent models have presented decreased, increased and unaltered PKC activity [146-148]. Studies of mesangial and smooth muscle cells have linked

PKC activation to diminished Na^+/K^+-ATPase function [149]. On the other hand, both PKC antagonists and agonists normalized Na^+/K^+ pumping in peripheral nerves of diabetic animals, suggesting a conflicting involvement of PKC enhancement and diminishment in the mechanism of Na^+/K^+-ATPase deficits [146]. It is thus intriguing how administration of a PKC-β selective inhibitor, LY333531, restored sciatic nerve blood flow and NCVs in STZ-induced diabetes [150, 151]. In addition, little data from humans, if any, has been obtained to support a PKC change in diabetic peripheral nerves. These experimental results nonetheless implicated PKC inhibition as a prospective avenue for anti-diabetic complication to investigators. The same inhibitor LY333531 (by Eli Lily) with a generic name Ruboxistaurin entered clinical evaluation as a treatment for DPN. In the trial of a small cohort of patients, Vinik *et al* reported that a 32 mg/day Ruboxistaurin for 6 months elicited significant alleviation on skin microvascular blood flow, total sensory symptoms and quality of life [152]. Recently, a 18-week treatment of Ruboxistaurin to a smaller subset of patients with type 2 diabetes proved beneficial in improving total symptom score (NTSS-6) and quality of life [153]. Unfortunately, this did not translate to a multinational, randomized, phase II, double-blind, placebo-controlled study consisting of 205 patients at an equal or double dosage of Ruboxistaurin [154]. Although Ruboxistaurin is well tolerated, Eli Lily withdrew its marketing authorization application.

2.3. Increasing neurotrophic support

2.3.1. Growth factors and growth factor replacement therapy

Mammalian nervous system depends on a group of endogenous and heterogeneous biomolecules for proper physiological functions including growth, survival, differentiation and regeneration. Nerve growth factor (NGF), brain-derived neurotrophic factor (BDNF) and neurotrophin-3 (NT-3) from the neurotrophin family are retrogradely transported to neuronal cell bodies after secretion from organs innervated by nerve terminals. These three neurotrophins regulate the activity of small nociceptive and sympathetic sensory fibers, medium size sensory and motor fibers, large diameter sensorimotor and sympathetic neurons, respectively [155]. Other frequently studied growth factors in this context are glial-derived neurotrophic factor (GDNF), ciliary neurotrophic factor (CNTF) as well as insulin-like growth factor-1 (IGF-1), which are expressed by peripheral glia and/or neurons and manifest diverse trophic effects on sensory, motor and autonomic nerves [156]. In experimental rodent models, the protein and/or mRNA levels of NGF, BDNF and NT-3 have been observed to both upregulate and downregulate in peripheral nerves, sensory glia and such target tissues as skin keratinocytes, skeletal muscles and submandibular glands [157-164]. Despite these conflicting reports, it is generally believed that the retrograde and anterograde axonal transport of these neurotrophins are diminished in diabetic nerves [14, 165]. Similarly, IGF-1 and CNTF were found to be reduced in various tissues examined in type 1 and type 2 diabetic rat models [166-168]. In STZ or diabetic BB/Wor rats, deficient NGF and IGF-1 level correlated with inadequate macrophage recruitment and Wallerian degeneration after sciatic nerve injury [166, 169]. As postulated by the authors and others, this may explain the perturbed nerve regeneration in diabetes. Considering the highly dynamic nerve degeneration/regeneration in the initial stage of DPN, growth factor therapy early in disease progression may minimize the damage and aid the axonal repair. To this end, abundant support has been produced using an array of spontaneous, chemical or transgenic diabetic models administered recombinant growth factors. Of note, NGF treatment restored neuropeptide level, C-fiber function and dermal myelinated innervation, alleviated neuropathic pain and promoted injury repair [156]. Whereas BDNF and NT-3 elicited a preferential attenuation in the structural and functional changes of large myelinated sensory and motor fibers [14], GDNF and IGF-1 showed a broad preservation of somatic and autonomic nervous system [19, 156]. Moreover, CNTF administration prevented/rescued behavioral and electrophysiological dysfunction, and enhanced sensory nerve resprouting in rats previously injected STZ [168, 170].

In humans, there is no prevailing trend of change in the serum level of NGF in type 2 cohorts with symptomatic DPN [171, 172]. Another study revealed significantly weaker immunoreactivity of NGF in the lateral calf skin of a group of type 1 diabetics who presented with asymptomatic, early length-dependent loss of nociception and axon reflex vasodilation [173]. However, analysis of the same site from a mixed population of type 1 and type 2 patients with mild early neuropathy indicated that expression of NGF transcripts was higher compared to healthy individuals [174]. Furthermore, epidermal NT-3 protein level markedly increased as a function of the severity of diabetic polyneuropathy [175], whereas CNTF did not vary in postmortem sciatic nerve autopsies between normal and DPN subjects [176]. Likewise, sural nerve IGF-1 mRNA expression was not altered by different durations of DPN [177]. Differing from the findings in animal nerves [161, 178], diabetic humans who developed neuropathy express more trkA and trkC, specific receptors for NGF and NT-3, in the epidermis than those without neuropathy [179]. Whether this reflects a tissue-specific response to diabetes awaits further examination of human nerve biopsies. Clinical testing of recombinant human NGF (rhNGF) perhaps witnessed one of the most spectacular failures in DPN trials. A phase II trial on 250 patients for 6 months reported a robust amelioration on subjective and objective sensory measurements, particularly the components related to small fiber sensory function [180]. When proceeded to a large-scale, multicenter,1-year phase III trial, 1019 participants randomized to receive either placebo or subcutaneous injection of rhNGF could not confirm a neuroprotective effect [181]. Most importantly, severe painful side effects including injection site hyperalgesia and diffuse myalgia significantly limited the tolerable dose to less than 1μg/kg, a dosage 1000 times lower than most of those used in experimental models. This contradicts preclinical data from rodents in which application of NGF reduced pain thresholds [156, 182]. On the opposite side, the observation that NGF evokes pain or hypersensitivity in both animals and humans led to the conception that anti-NGF therapy may reduce neuropathic pain [183-185]. This appeared to be the case in a variety of chronic inflammatory and cancer pain models in which hyperalgesia and/or allodynia were effectively attenuated by antibodies blocking NGF or TrkA [186-188]. In this regard, some proof-of-concept, positive results have been generated in a recent phase III trial on osteoarthritis for a monoclonal antibody against NGF (tanezumab) [189]. However, Pfizer had to temporarily suspend the studies involving DPN after disease worsening and joint replacements occurred in the treatment group.

Other than NGF, a double-blind, placebo-controlled study was also conducted for rhBDNF but found no evidence of improvements on the primary endpoints associated with diabetic sensory neuropathy [190]. Although rhGDNF and rhNT-3 were supposed to enter early clinical assessments for DPN management, they have not yielded any clinical report except the withdrawal of NT-3 from phase I study [156]. It is therefore apparent that the expected outcomes were not met. For IGF-1 and CNTF, development of replacement therapy is also hindered by their non-specific impacts on the central nervous system [191] and muscles [192], respectively.

2.4. Modulating neurovascular function

2.4.1. Nerve blood flow and angiotensin-converting enzyme inhibitors

Multiple epidemiological analyses have previously identified that hypertension strongly increases the occurrence and severity of DPN in population studies [1]. Spontaneously hypertensive diabetic rats developed a more severe behavioral, physiological and structural phenotype pertinent to clinical DPN [193]. Tissues of neuropathic diabetic patients manifest augmented vasoconstrictive response and diminuted endoneurial blood flow [194]. In turn, vascular deficiency and impaired peripheral nerve perfusion contribute to neural hypoxia and ischemia, two of the well-recognized factors in the pathogenesis of microvascular complications in diabetes. This provides a rationale for enhancing vasodilation as a treatment regimen in counteracting diabetes-induced neurovascular stress. This assumption is backed by the observations in experimental diabetes that motor and sensory conduction deficits were normalized by several vasodilating agents with distinct pharmacological actions [195-197]. The most well-established class of compounds in this scenario is angiotensin-converting enzyme (ACE) inhibitors. ACE inhibitors stimulate endothelium-dependent release of nitric oxide and vessel relaxation by antagonizing ACE-mediated formation of the potent vasoconstrictor angiotensin II and deactivation of bradykinin, a strong vasodilator [198]. Combination of these hypotensive effects by ACE inhibitors corrected reductions in nerve blood flow, capillary densities and conduction measurements in STZ-induced diabetic or Zucker fatty rats [199-201].

Although ACE inhibitors are the first line treatment for nephropathy and cardiovascular condition in diabetes [202], there is scarce evidence suggesting the same for diabetic neuropathy. To date, only one small double-blinded, randomized, placebo-controlled DPN clinical study has been conducted on one ACE inhibitor, trandalapril [203]. In this study, normotensive DPN patients treated with trandalapril over 1 year demonstrated significant improvements in electrophysiological function but not QST, neuropathy symptom/deficit score or autonomic function. A major disappointment came from the Appropriate Blood Pressure Control in Diabetes (ABCD) trial. This prospective study followed 470 type 2 diabetic patients for 5.3 years and found neither moderate nor intensive blood pressure control using nisoldipine (Ca^{2+} blocker) or enalapril (ACE inhibitor) was effective in modulating the progression of diabetic triopathy (neuropathy, nephropathy, retinopathy) [204]. Furthermore, there were no overall differential outcomes between interventions. This result along with the fact that clinical

DPN develops and exacerbates in many patients that regularly take the ACE inhibitor casts reasonable doubt on the extent to which ACE intervention is useful in DPN management [205].

2.4.2. *Vascular supply and vascular endothelial growth factor therapy*

Another approach to address vascular insufficiency is to promote the angiogenesis via expression of vascular endothelial growth factor (VEGF), a cytokine primarily mitogenic for vascular endothelial cells. Overexpression of VEGF through gene transfer stimulated vascularization in both animals [206, 207] and humans [208, 209]. Diabetes was shown to compromise the expression of this growth factor in the skin of patients who also had loss of intraepidermal nerve fiber density (IENFD) [210]. In comparison, most evidence derived from diabetic rodents contradicts with this finding and indicates an upregulation of VEGF in diabetic tissues [211] thatcan be normalized by insulin or NGF infusion [212]. If these observations are true, this could mean VEGF is differentially involved in the pathogenetic processes underlying human and rodent DPN. It is paradoxical, however, that preliminary studies using the same models in which pathological VEGF induction by diabetes was seen also generated data favoring VEGF-enhancing gene therapy in treating DPN. For example, subcutaneous inoculation of herpes simplex virus carrying VEGF-transgene in STZ rats prevented multiple characteristics of experimental DPN, particularly those associated with dorsal sensory function [213]. In a separate report, intramuscular delivery of plasmid DNA encoding VEGF-1 or VEGF-2 completely reversed attenuation of nerve blood flow, slowing of NCV, destruction of vasa nervorum, and dysfunction of small and large fibers in STZ rats [214]. The same study was also able to reproduce the results in rabbits with alloxan-induced diabetes. Two randomized controlled trials (RCTs) have been undertaken to translate this experimental approach to clinical usage. The first trial tested intramuscular VEGF-1 or VEGF-2 gene transfer in 50 DPN patients with presenting symptoms of pain and/or numbness, and achieved an improvement on symptom score, regions of sensory loss and visual analog pain scale over 6-month duration [215]. Other primary and secondary endpoints including quantitative sensory and electrophysiological testing were not met. In addition, there were significantly more severe adverse events in gene therapy group compared to placebo group. Among the listed events, hemorrhage, diabetic retinopathy and peripheral edema had been previously brought up as concerns but apparently were not properly addressed during preclinical animal evaluation [216]. The second trial was reported in a published meeting presentation by Sangamo BioSciences, which announced the phase I/II results for a series of injectable plasmids encoding VEGF gene-targeting zinc-finger DNA-binding transcription factor with proven-efficacy in experimental models [217]. Of these, SB-509 was praised to be well-tolerated with a most positive outcome in sensory nerve conduction velocity (SNCV), IENFD and neuropathic impairment score. However, the treatment arm as a whole did not obtain a convincing benefit versus placebo to make this a successful trial. With an argument by Sangamo that a carefully chosen cohort may be more sensitive to SB-509, a latest phase IIb study was set to recruit 170 patients with moderate or severe DPN. Despite broad outcome measures and rigorous analysis, the trial was concluded as being unequivocally disappointing which led to the eventual cessation of this Sangamo's lead program [218].

2.4.3. Lipid metabolism and γ-linolenic acid

γ-Linolenic acid is an important precursor for arachidonic acid. The latter produces the potent vasodilator and platelet inhibitor prostacyclin or prostaglandin I_2 (PGI_2) [219], lack of which can increase the risk of developing thrombosis in diabetic vessels [24] and microvascular diseases. γ-Linolenic acid is primarily synthesized from the dietary ω-6 essential fatty acid linolenic acid, but this reaction is impaired in STZ or alloxan-treated rats [220, 221]. In human type 1 diabetic patients, disturbed fatty acid metabolism has also been inferred from the serum lipid profile [222, 223]. Since γ-linolenic acid also forms the neuronal phospholipids [224, 225], direct supplementation of this polyunsaturated fatty acid can theoretically treat DPN by enhancing both microcirculation and membranous structures in the nervous system, such as the myelin. In keeping with this hypothesis, administration of γ-linolenic acid prevents or reverses the development of experimental DPN in rodents [226-229]. Clinical assessments of the evening primrose oil, the herbal source of γ-linolenic acid, took place in the United Kingdom and suggested an efficacious treatment effect on human DPN [230, 231]. However, some negative outcomes have been obtained for γ-linolenic acid in other clinical conditions by independent groups [232, 233] and the British General Medical Counsel filed a report that the efficacy of evening primrose oil in diabetics claimed by one company-funded trial was falsified [234]. Some issues related to marketing fraud and publication suppression by the drug company attempting to develop evening primrose oil for clinical use have also been raised [235, 236]. Due to these controversies, UK's Medicines Control Agency withdrew the drug's product license. As of today, no further evidence has been acquired to confirm the validity of γ-linolenic acid as an anti-DPN medicine.

2.5. Counteracting oxidative stress

2.5.1. Reactive oxygen species and α-lipoic acid

After years of investigations through experimental approaches which harvested knowledge on a plethora of biochemical pathways linking hyperglycemic stress to nerve injury, a general consensus has been reached by the DPN research community that all these complex molecular and cellular events converge on and interact with one universal consequence, oxidative stress [45, 237]. Direct and indirect evidence of oxidative stress in tissue sites of diabetic complications is overwhelming in animals with induced diabetes. In general, hyperglycemia induces a composite oxidative insult to neurons, SCs as well as vasa nervorum through: 1) accelerated free radicals production; 2) increased oxidation and nitration of proteins, lipids and nucleic acids; and 3) deprivation of antioxidant defense system [238]. Many excellent reviews have illustrated and discussed the pathophysiological consequences of redox imbalance in the peripheral nervous system (PNS) [45, 239] therefore an elaborated description will not be provided here. Briefly, increased intracellular glucose metabolism through the classical glycolytic tricarboxylic acid cycle leads to mitochondrial nutrient overload and subsequently uncontrolled superoxide (O_2^-) production by its oxidative respiratory machinery. Excessive generation of superoxide in conjunction with polyol synthesis exhausts the detoxificating agents including superoxide dismutase and GSH. This eventually gives rise to accumulation of other reactive oxygen (ROS) and nitrogen species (RNS) such as hydrogen peroxide (H_2O_2), hydroxyl radicals (OH•) and peroxynitrite (NO•). Other hyperglycemia-initiated events such as AGE formation and NGF deficiency have also been suggested to fuel the ROS generation in various compartments. These highly reactive free radicals can non-specifically oxidize and nitrosylate cellular/extracellular biomolecules and undermine organellar function. Particularly, increased protein nitration, lipid peroxidation products and mitochondria dysfunction are predominant phenomena in DRGs and sciatic nerves in diabetic animals [240-242]. Compared to the clear evidence of oxidative damage in experimental DPN, expression of the correspondent biomarkers indicating oxidative stress in human tissues is rather vague [239, 243]. Some studies even suggested a reduced free radical reaction in diabetic patients versus normal control [244, 245]. Further, despite a strong rationale and the promise of substantial neuroprotection by anti-oxidant treatments in rodent diabetics [246-249], this anti-oxidative approach is not spared from the irreproducibility of the results obtained from basic research in clinical practice.

Among a number of anti-oxidants that corrected experimental DPN, α-lipoic acid (ALA) has gone the furthest into clinical use, while the others have proven largely ineffective [14, 250]. ALA or thioctic acid is naturally synthesized in mitochondria and has a powerful antioxidant capacity because of its dual ability to scavenge ROS/transition metals and regenerate other endogenous antioxidants. Approximately 7 double-masked multicenter RCTs, including the series of ALADIN, SYDNEY and NATHAN, testing the efficacy of ALA in treating symptomatic DPN have been completed in Europe [251]. Of these, a general benefit on sensory symptoms and deficits was extrapolated by a meta-analysis incorporating 4 trials (ALADIN I, ALADIN III, SYDNEY, NATHAN II) that treated subjects with 600 mg/day ALA via intravenous infusion for 3 weeks [252]. However, there is an overall mixed bag of results and several therapeutically important indices including symptoms score, nerve conduction and QST were not consistently ameliorated in these studies [205, 252, 253]. Notably, some asserted improvement fell below the clinically meaningful threshold of 30% when adjusted to placebo control [254]. It is also discouraging that trials in which patients received oral dosing of ALA presented only marginal benefit; this significantly precludes the oral application of ALA. Although ALA has been marketed in Germany for treating DPN and is available as nutritional supplement in the US, current existing evidence suggests that ALA at best only retards the neuropathic progression in diabetes.

3. Scientific rationale for the limited translational success: What have we learned?

Based on the records published by National Institute of Neurological Disorders and Stroke (NINDS), a main source of DPN research, about 16,488 projects were funded at the expense of over $8 billion for the fiscal years of 2008 through 2012. Of these projects, an estimated 72,200 animals were used annually to understand basic physiology and disease pathology as well as to evaluate potential drugs [255]. As discussed above, however, the usefulness of these pharmaceutical agents developed through such a pipeline in preventing or reducing neuronal damage has been equivocal and usually halted at human trials due to toxicity, lack of efficacy or both (Figure 1). Clearly, the pharmacological translation from our decades of experimental modeling to clinical practice with regard to DPN has thus far not even close to satisfactory. Undoubtedly, the flawed design of some clinical trials has led to the inadequate evaluation of certain candidate compounds and for a thorough discussion on this specific topic the readers are referred elsewhere [256]. In this section, we focus on discussing some of the fundamental species differences that render a direct translation unrealistic.

3.1. Failure to predict toxic effects

Whereas a majority of the drugs investigated during preclinical testing executed experimentally desired endpoints without revealing significant toxicity, more than half that entered clinical evaluation for treating DPN were withdrawn as a consequence of moderate to severe adverse events even at a much lower dose. Generally, using other species as surrogates for human population inherently encumbers the accurate prediction of toxic reactions for several reasons.

First of all, it is easy to dismiss drug-induced non-specific effects in animals—especially for laboratory rodents who do not share the same size, anatomy and physical activity with humans. Events such as cardiac attack are often overlooked without a complex and careful examination. A case in point is the anti-diabetic drug Avandia for which the market approval has been a center of dispute. Avandia's active ingredient rosiglitazone promotes insulin sensitivity by activating peroxisome proliferator-activated receptors (PPARs) and was claimed by its maker GlaxoSmithKline to be safe in the preclinical report. Some even went further to advocate the favorable application of rosiglitazone to heart conditions based on its positive influence on cardiovascular biomarkers in rodent studies [257, 258]. Only after accumulating incidents of congestive heart failure among patients receiving Avandia was presented to the FDA, did it begin to spur wide concerns and active investigations of the serious cardiotoxicity by Avandia in humans and animals [259].

Second, some physiological and behavioral phenotypes observable in humans are impossible for animals to express. In this aspect, photosensitive skin rash and pain serve as two good examples of non-translatable side effects. Rodent skin differs from that of humans in that it has a thinner and hairier epidermis and distinct DNA repair abilities [260]. Therefore, most rodent stains used in diabetes modeling provide poor estimates for the probability of cutaneous hypersensitivity reactions to pharmacological treatments [261]. Although skin engraftment onto nude mice has been attempted to circumvent this issue [260], mice with immunodeficiency do not constitute an appropriate background for studying diabetes. Another predicament is to assess pain in rodents. The reason for this is simple: these animals cannot tell us when, where or even whether they are experiencing pain, leaving us to read. Since there is not any specific type of behavior to which painful reaction can be unequivocally associated, this often leads to underestimation of painful side effects during preclinical drug screening (e.g. rhNGF).

The third problem is that animals and humans have different pharmacokinetic and toxicological responses. For instance, troglitazone (Rezulin), another anti-hyperglycemic PPAR agonist, was withdrawn after inducing idiosyncratic liver failure in patients but a similar hepatotoxicity could not be reproduced in animal models [262, 263]. Even in organ systems that were previously defined as having an overall high rate of interspecies toxicity concordance, unanticipated drug toxicity can still occur. This was the case for trastuzumab (Herceptin), a humanized monoclonal antibody that treats advanced breast carcinoma by binding and blocking human epidermal growth factor receptor 2 (HER2). Both preclinical and on-going toxicological studies in rhesus monkeys and rodents indicated no evidence of cardiac dysfunction [264]. However, trastuzumab administration to patients during clinical trials caused frequent and severe cardiomyopathy [265]. As discussed in a published scientific document of Herceptin toxicity by the European Medicines Agency, it is also unsuitable to assess the cytotoxicity of this antibody that specifically recognizes a single human protein in nonhuman species which have a distinct molecular and immunogenic environment [264]. In addition to the inaccuracies, disparities in pharmacokinetics underpin some of the extreme species differences. MPTP (1-methyl-4-phenyl-1,2,3,6-tetrahydropyridine)-induced neurotoxicity is a classic example. MPTP becomes poisonous to dopaminergic neurons once metabolized to MPP^+ by the enzyme monoamine oxidase-B (MAO-B) and elicits permanent Parkinson-like symptoms in human subjects [266]. In sharp contrast, MPTP is barely psychoactive in rats since they produce minimal MPP^+ and only mild damage to mouse brains due to much faster clearance of MPP^+ compared to primates [267]. By the same token, 350 mg of aspirin can be eliminated by half from human circulation in about 3 hours but retained in feline plasma for 37.5 hours, which is essentially lethal to these animals [268]. The argument can be finally strengthened by the work of two independent groups, who compared bioavailability between primates, rodents and dogs for various drugs and both demonstrated that no correlation exists between animal and human data [269]. The matter of drug-induced non-specific effects and uniquely human phenotypes may theoretically be resolved via rigorous pathological evaluation and better experimental method. By comparison, the pharmacokinetic and toxicological data highlights profound interspecies barriers and may not succumb to current technical manipulation. Considering some of the drugs were withdrawn when unexpected toxicological outcomes occur in only 1-2% of the population, relying on laboratory models to predict drug safety certainly puts us in a dilemma with very little medical and ethical risks from which our society can suffer (Figure 1).

3.2. Failure to recapitulate human neuropathologies

Genetic or chemical-induced diabetic rats or mice have been a major tool for preclinical pharmacological evaluation of potential DPN treatments. Yet, they do not faithfully reproduce many neuropathological manifestations in human diabetics. The difficulty of such begins with the fact that it is not possible to obtain in rodents a qualitative and quantitative expression of the clinical symptoms that are frequently presented in neuropathic diabetic patients, including spontaneous pain of different characteristics (e.g. prickling, tingling, burning, squeezing), paresthesia and numbness. As symptomatic changes constitute an important parameter of therapeutic outcome, this may well underlie the failure of some aforementioned drugs in clinical trials despite their good performance in experimental tests measuring behavioral responses of animals to external stimuli (Table 1). Development of nerve dysfunction in diabetic rodents also does not follow the common natural history of human DPN. As described earlier, sensory neuropathy in humans typically adopts a length-dependent, "stocking-glove" loss of sensation that slowly progresses from distal to proximal. Such a pattern was never functionally recapitulated in the commonly used type 1 and type 2 diabetic animal models, including STZ-injected rats, Zucker diabetic fatty (ZDF) rats and db/db mice. Besides the lack of anatomical resemblance, the changes in disease severity are often missing in these models. For example, although the majority of diabetic rodent models developed thermal hypoalgesia with long durations of diabetes as revealed by the sensory assay correspondent to that of QSTs in humans, there is no agreement between different studies in a consistent trend of progressive decline in thermal pain perception [270-272], a well-known phenomenon in patients. Alterations in thermal sensation in the tails of diabetic rodents varied upon studies and species used [273-275] and several groups have documented increased temperature perception after prolonged diabetes [276, 277], thus falsifying the relevance of tail flick test to human conditions. More importantly, foot ulcers that occur as a late complication to 15% of all individuals with diabetes [14] do not spontaneously develop in hyperglycemic rodents. Superimposed injury by experimental procedure in the foot pads of diabetic rats or mice may lend certain insight in the impaired wound healing in diabetes [278] but is not reflective of the chronic, accumulating pathological changes in diabetic feet of human counterparts. Another salient feature of human DPN that has not been described in animals is the predominant sensory and autonomic nerve damage versus minimal involvement of motor fibers [279]. This should elicit particular caution as the selective susceptibility is critical to our true understanding of the etiopathogenesis underlying distal sensorimotor polyneuropathy in diabetes. In addition to the lack of specificity, most animal models studied only cover a narrow spectrum of clinical DPN and have not successfully duplicated syndromes including proximal motor neuropathy and focal lesions [279].

Morphologically, fiber atrophy and axonal loss exist in STZ-rats and other diabetic rodents but are much milder compared to the marked degeneration and loss of myelinated and unmyelinated nerves readily observed in human specimens [280]. Of significant note, rodents are notoriously resistant to developing some of the histological hallmarks seen in diabetic patients, such as segmental and paranodal demyelination [44]. There are sporadic reports of demyelination in STZ and genetically diabetic Bio-Breeding (BB) rats after 8-12 months of diabetes [58, 281-283]. However, this is apparently related to a different microvascular pathology as morphometric analysis of sural and tibial vasa nervorum in these rats revealed dilated lumina, flattening of endothelial cells and microvessel walls [284], contrasting with the basement membrane thickening, endothelial hyperplagia and narrowing of endoneurial lumen in human diabetics [285, 286]. Similarly, the simultaneous presence of degenerating and regenerating fibers that is characteristic of early DPN has not been clearly demonstrated in these animals [44]. Since such dynamic nerve degeneration/regeneration signifies an active state of nerve repair and is most likely to be amenable to therapeutic intervention, absence of this property makes rodent models a poor tool in both deciphering disease pathogenesis and designing treatment approaches. Given that our ability to devise a cure for human DPN depends ultimately on our successful understanding and reduction of its various functional and structural indexes, failure of most animal models to replicate these human neuropathologies with high fidelity renders this task difficult at best.

Species/ Models Characteristics	Humans	Induced		Spontaneous				Transgenic/ Knockout mice
		STZ-rats/mice	BB/Wor-rats	NOD mice	ZDF rats	ob/ob mice	db/db mice	
Disease Genesis	multigenic	monogenic						
Onset	chronic (years to decades)	acute (3 days)	moderate (2-5 months)	unpredictable (4-30 weeks)	mild (1-2 months)			various, superimposed by other diabetogenic protocols
Progression	slow, chronic (years to decades)	Rapid (6-20 weeks)				Slow (11-68 weeks)		
Glycemic Profile	moderate hyperglycemia	severe hyperglycemia	severe/fatal hyperglycemia, requires insulin for life preservation		severe hyperglycemia	normo- to mild hyper-glycemia	moderate hyperglycemia	
Symptoms	varying degree and properties of pain, paresthesia, numbness, insensitivity, absent reflexes, muscle weakness	no clear definition/presentation of spontaneous pain or other symptoms; thermal/mechanical hyperalgesia and tactile allodynia are often used as indication of increased pain perception however cannot be differentiated from increased sensory function						
Sensory Function	thermal hypoalgesia, decreased vibration perception threshold, loss of Achilles reflex	mechanical hyperalgesia, thermal hyperalgesia/hypoalgesia, mechanical/tactile allodynia	thermal hyperalgesia	thermal hyperalgesia/ hypoalgesia, tactile allodynia	thermal/ mechanical hyperalgesia	thermal/ mechanical hypoalgesia	thermal hypoalgesia	various
Nerve Conduction	progressive decrease at a rate of 0.5m/s per year	>10m/s reduction within 6-20 weeks						
Morphology	loss of unmyelinated and myelinated fibers, evidence of axonal degeneration and regeneration, segmental and paranodal demyelination, distal axonotrophy; basement membrane thickening, narrowing of endoneuriallumina	distal axonotrophy, myelinated fiber atrophy, few axonal loss, demyelination only after long-term hyperglycemia; basement membrane flattening, widening of microvascularlumina		axonal atrophy and degeneration	not characterized	slight fiber atrophy and loss; basement membrane thickening, narrowing of endoneuriallumina		various
Nerve Biochemistry	sorbitol, fructose content not altered or slightly elevated, much lower compared to rodents at both healthy and diabetic states; myo-inositol level unchanged	sorbitol, fructose level highly increased by diabetes; myo-inositol level markedly reduced		unclear		sorbitol, fructose level normal or moderately elevated; myo-inositol level unchanged		AR-overexpressing mice exhibit exaggerated increase of polyol pathway metabolites and reduction of myo-inositol
Overall Limitation of the Model		phenotypic exaggeration and acceleration driven mostly by severe hyperglycemia				representing early or prediabetesrather than overt diabetes		amplifying specific components, applicable to rare cases

Abbreviations: NOD=non-obese diabetic, AR=aldose reductase

Table 1. Comparison of DPN Characteristics between Humans and Frequently Used Laboratory Rodent Models

3.3. Overrepresentation of pathogenetic pathways

STZ is a glucose analog of selective toxicity to pancreatic β-cells and induces insulin-deficiency and hyperglycemia mimicking that in human type 1 diabetes mellitus. Injection of this chemical provides a convenient and affordable tool in inducing robust hyperglycemia in animals with good control over disease onset and duration. Therefore, STZ-rats have been favored by researchers during preclinical drug assessments for diabetic complications [280]. However, STZ typically produces a rather immediate, severe hypoinsulinemia and elevation of blood glucose, whereas the development of hyperglycemia in most human conditions is slow and modest [287]. The contrariety manifests stably in the serum HbA1c levels. While the non-diabetic range (~4-5.6%) is similar, a single administration of STZ to Wistar rats can increase the HbA1c to above 12% in 4-5 weeks [288, 289], which indicates a very poor glucose control that is considered rare in the clinic setting with anti-diabetic care. In fact, less than 15% of patients may have an HbA1c level exceeding 9% by sample estimation [290]. Such extreme hyperglycemia in STZ-treated rats could give rise to exaggerated glucose accumulation and metabolic derangements that would not be commonly present in human diabetics. Indeed, the concentrations of sorbitol and fructose per unit weight of nerve tissue in STZ diabetic rats is consistently increased and dramatically higher in comparison with human diabetics, who on average also do not uniformly show upregulation of these glucose metabolites via polyol pathway [44, 55, 79]. Of interesting note, under normal physiological conditions the contents of nerve sorbitol in rodents are almost 10-fold higher than those in humans, suggesting some species difference in the relative involvement of AR in glucose metabolism during both normo- and hyperglycemia. Observations of polyol pathway utilization in different species and cell types vary widely; the total glucose utilization through polyol pathway is one third in rabbit ocular lenses and only one tenth in human erythrocytes in response to high glucose stress [45, 291]. Consistent with an inverse association between increased polyol flux and electrophysiological dysfunction, diabetic rodents frequently exhibit 10 m/s or more reduction in NCV within the typical 6-20 week experimental duration [271, 292-294]. By contrast, the deterioration of NCV in human patients gradually takes place and has an average loss of 0.5 m/s per year [1] (Table 1). It is also suspicious that the profound and precipitated NCV deceleration in STZ-rodents occur without apparent histopathological changes, which can be a prominent feature in diabetic neuropathic patients at early stage. Therefore, enhanced AR activity might contribute differently or less significantly to the pathogenesis of DPN in humans than rodents. This could explain why AR inhibitors, and by extension, many other pathogenetically targeted inhibitors afford potent neuroprotection in experimental studies but only marginal effects in clinical trials.

Another criticism is that most STZ models were rendered diabetic at puberty since administering STZ to rodents after sexual maturation cannot always produce peripheral nerve abnormalities [280, 295]. Unlike matured nerves that displayed little change in response to diabetic insults, immature peripheral nerves readily manifest hyperglycemia-induced morphological and electrophysiological deficits within an even shorter duration [295]. However, such a phenotype bears little relevance to 90% of clinical conditions, in which diabetes-induced nerve damage has an adult onset and slow time course.

3.4. Other physical and environmental factors

Humans certainly share considerable biological similarities with other mammals. In the nervous system, these include some of the nociceptive responses and higher cognitive activities. At the same time, no one would suggest that humans and animals are the same—they obviously differ in many physiological and behavioral aspects. The question is: can we obtain effective therapeutic applicability after evolution has well separated our species from others? In order to answer this, it is necessary to carefully examine these differences and their impacts on the pharmacokinetic and pharmacological extrapolation. As delineating every single molecular, cellular and phenotypic difference is a laborious task, we will highlight only those relevant to our discussion of DPN. When comparing humans with the conventionally used experimental animals, namely rats and mice, the most conspicuous difference is anatomical. With particular respect to neuroanatomy, a peripheral axon in humans can reach as long as one meter [296] whereas the maximal length of the axons innervating the hind limb is five centimeters in mice and twelve centimeters in rats. This short length makes it impossible to study in rodents the prominent length dependency and dying-back feature of peripheral nerve dysfunction that characterizes human DPN. Even if size were an issue and macro-structure appears similar, there might still be striking differences in the micro-structure within the tissue or organ. This is the case for insulin-secreting islets. For decades the cytoarchitecture of human islets was assumed to be just like those in rodents with a clear anatomical subdivision of β-cells and other cell types. By using confocal microscopy and multi-fluorescent labeling, it was finally uncovered that human islets have not only a substantially lower percentage of β-cell population, but also a mixed—rather than compartmentalized—organization of the different cell types [297]. This cellular arrangement was demonstrated to directly alter the functional performance of human islets as opposed to rodent islets. Although it is not known whether such profound disparities in cell composition and association also exist in the PNS, it might as well be anticipated considering the many sophisticated sensory and motor activities that are unique to humans.

Considerable species difference also manifest at a molecular level. The chemical structure and signaling profile of a molecule may not always be conserved throughout the evolution. Such difference, although small, can account for a significant translational limitation for pharmacological treatments targeted at a specific biomolecule. A good explanation is the case of trastuzumab. As mentioned earlier, trastuzumab was specifically designed to immuno-antagonize HER2, thereby inhibiting cancer cell growth. However, this drug could not be adequately assessed in rodents or primates because of the inability of this human protein-targeting antibody to recognize the HER2 homologues expressed in these nonhuman species [264]. Despite the successful employment of nude mice for the preclinical evaluation of trastuzumab, a comprehensive pharmacological and pharmacokinetic profile was not obtained for this humanized antibody and it resulted in unpredicted toxicity in patients. While the molecular difference might not be as serious of a problem for rhNGF and rhVEGF, critical retrospective examination into this aspect may lend some insight into the failure of these gene therapies in DPN trials. At least 80% of human genes have a counterpart in the mouse and rat genome. However, temporal and spatial expression of these genes can vary remarkably between humans and rodents, in terms of both extent and isoform specificity. The first is evident from the differential level of MAO-B expression in humans and rats which resulted in distinct susceptibility of these two species to MPTP-induced neurotoxicity [266]. The second category involves protein families comprising multiple isoforms owing to different promoter usage and alternative gene splicing. For instance, the enzyme PKC has at least 12 different subtypes, of which, PKC-α is predominantly expressed in human hearts and PKC-ε in rodents [298]. Since activation of PKC-α and PKC-ε are differentially regulated, species-specific PKC inhibitors will need to be developed in order to efficiently block the pathogenic action of this kinase in cardiomyopathy, especially when a non-selective inhibition of PKC function is unwanted or even detrimental. Given that the efficacy of ruboxistaurin in treating DPN was also based on data from rat diabetic models [150, 151], it is imperative to speculate that the unsatisfactory results of ruboxistaurin in patients is due at least in part to a relatively less important role of PKC-β in the pathological development of diabetic human nerves. The last type of molecular difference is that the components along a particular signaling axis may be preferentially vulnerable to pathological alteration in different species. This possibility has been largely ignored but could underpin a major limitation in current translational research. One typical example is that much has been learned regarding the anti-hyperphagic effects of leptin from ob/ob mice, which also led to the exciting finding that administration of this hormone can successfully suppress weight gain [299]. Nonetheless, this offered little treatment benefit for the majority of obese people (99.95%) who have impaired signaling downstream of leptin instead of leptin deficiency as observed in ob/ob mice [300]. Some may argue that these issues can be overcome by creating genetically engineered or "humanized" mice in which a mouse gene is substituted by the human version. However, transgenic or knockout mice can be afflicted with developmental deficits and alterations which are inappropriate for modeling a chronic disease that appears in the later life time, such as type 2 diabetes and its complications. Moreover, we do not know whether a genetically introduced human protein—if it is different enough from the murine orthologue that a transgene is necessary—faithfully maintains the same expression and interaction properties in mouse system as it would in humans.

Ultimately, a fundamental problem associated with resorting to rodents in DPN research is to study a human disorder that takes decades to develop and progress in organisms with a maximum lifespan of 2-3 years. The longest duration of experimental diabetes in a rodent model was documented by Ras *et al.*, who observed leptin-deficient db/db mice for 17 months and reported only mild pathological changes in the peripheral nerve fibers [301]. It is thus fair to say that a full clinical spectrum of the maturity-onset DPN likely requires a length of time exceeding the longevity of rodents to present and diabetic rodent models at best only help illustrate the very early aspects of the entire disease syndrome. Since none of the early pathogenetic pathways revealed in diabetic rodents will contribute to DPN in a quantitatively and temporally uniform fashion throughout the prolonged natural history of this disease, it is not surprising that a handful of inhibitors developed against these processes have not benefited patients with relatively long-standing neuropathy. As a matter of fact, any agents targeting single biochemical insults would be too little too late to treat a chronic neurological disorder with established nerve damage and pathogenetic heterogeneity (Figure 2). In DPN, such heterogeneity is the consequence of a complex interplay between genetic predisposition, physical characteristics, nutritional and other environmental factors. On the contrary, experimental rodents are maintained at a homogeneous genetic background. Genetic homogeneity becomes particularly apparent with the inbred strains and genetically engineered mice, making them more of a tool to elucidate the contribution of a specific component to disease development and less of a tool for an accurate prediction of the likelihood that a treatment will be effective for a general population. Apart from these internal factors, laboratory caged animals have an uniform dietary constitution, life cycle and environmental contact, therefore would not be exposed to the majority of the external risk factors otherwise incurred by individual patients, such as smoking and alcohol consumption [10]. Finally, humans have some unique behaviors that assume an integral part of DPN-associated complications but cannot be adopted by animals. This is perhaps the simplest reason why diabetic rodents are immune to gangrenous foot ulceration as upright walking has not evolved in these species.

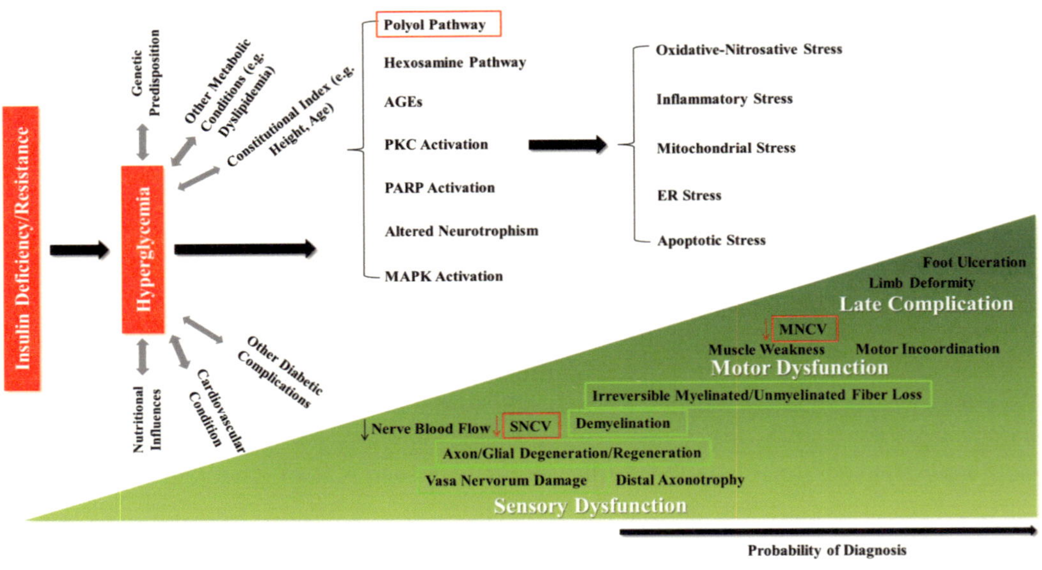

Figure 2. Schematic Demonstration of the Progressive Pathogenetic and Pathophysiological Changes in DPN. Components highlighted in red marks changes that are often over-exaggerated in frequently used rodent models, whereas those in green mark physiological and morphological changes not replicated or misreplicated. Darker color in the triangle box indicates less likely the pathologies are to be adequately modeled in rodents. Double-headed arrows indicate interaction. PARP: poly(ADP-ribose) polymerase, MAPK: mitogen-activated protein kinase, ER: endoplastic reticulum.

4. Conclusion and outlook

Needless to say, DPN has been a significant source of diabetes-induced mortality and morbidity that strike individuals, families and society with a staggering health and economic cost. There is little doubt that the need for effective DPN management is currently unmet and better therapeutic regimens ought to be sought. The invasive nature of present methods of biochemical, structural and functional measurements dictates that systemic and longitudinal assessments are not feasible in humans. To address this, miscellaneous rodent models have been created and used as substitutes for diabetic patients for the purpose of uncovering the pathogenetic mechanisms and testing potential pharmacological treatments. However, these conventional approaches have so far failed to yield a successful therapeutic translation. Further, animal surrogates are afflicted with species differences in genotype and behavior, nerve structure and metabolism, duration of diabetes, and tissue vulnerability, which allow limited transferability of animal results into clinical settings. It is important to point out that the present review does not argue against the ability of animal models to shed light on basic molecular, cellular and physiological processes that are shared among species. Undoubtedly, animal models of diabetes have provided abundant insights into the disease biology of DPN. Nevertheless, the lack of any meaningful advance in identifying a promising pharmacological target necessitates a reexamination of the validity of current DPN models as well as to offer a plausible alternative methodology to scientific approaches and disease intervention. After a critical reevaluation of the experimental results and clinical outcomes for several previously high-profile anti-DPN drugs, we conclude that the fundamental species differences have led to misinterpretation of rodent data and overall failure of pharmacological investment. As more is being learned, it is becoming prevailing that DPN is a chronic, heterogeneous disease unlikely to benefit from targeting specific and early pathogenetic components revealed by animal studies. Rather, an efficacious therapy must impact on multiple etiologic events and manage various risk factors. In this regard, rigorous lifestyle modulation may simultaneously intervene with a multitude of internal and external diabetogenic processes without generating significant tissue toxicity and side effects. Particularly, diet and exercise intervention provides an approach to improve metabolic management and enhance long-term reparative and regenerative capacity of diabetic nerves. Moreover, investigating the disease process via human-based study to the extent possible promises to lend much better insight into the pathology and pathogenesis of DPN as well as the clinical utility of potential treatments. We propose that future research should put an emphasis on advancing methodological and technological approaches that maximizes the access and utilization of human specimens under ethical guidelines, and on refining lifestyles for preventing and modifying DPN, which are more cost-effective and directly applicable to clinical practice in this otherwise largely intractable disorder.

Acknowledgements

This work is supported and funded by the Physicians Committee for Responsible Medicine. The authors thank Dr. Neal Barnard and Dr. Charu Chandrasekera for their help and expertise on this paper.

Author details

Chengyuan Li, Anne E. Bunner and John J. Pippin

Physicians Committee for Responsible Medicine, Washington, DC, USA

References

[1] Boulton AJ, Malik RA, Arezzo JC, Sosenko JM. Diabetic somatic neuropathies. Diabetes care. 2004;27(6):1458-86. Epub 2004/05/27.

[2] Vinik AI, Mehrabyan A. Diabetic neuropathies. The Medical clinics of North America. 2004;88(4):947-99, xi. Epub 2004/08/17.

[3] Dyck PJ. Detection, characterization, and staging of polyneuropathy: assessed in diabetics. Muscle & nerve. 1988;11(1):21-32. Epub 1988/01/01.

[4] Tesfaye S. Epidemiology and etiology of diabetic peripheral neuropathies. Adv Stud Med. 2004(4(suppl)):1014–20.

[5] Veves A, Backonja M, Malik RA. Painful diabetic neuropathy: epidemiology, natural history, early diagnosis, and treatment options. Pain Med. 2008;9(6):660-74. Epub 2008/10/02.

[6] Harati Y. Diabetic peripheral neuropathies. Methodist DeBakey cardiovascular journal. 2010;6(2):15-9. Epub 2010/07/28.

[7] Martyn CN, Hughes RA. Epidemiology of peripheral neuropathy. J Neurol Neurosurg Psychiatry. 1997;62(4):310-8. Epub 1997/04/01.

[8] Wild S RG, Green A, Sicree R, King H. Global prevalence of diabetes estimates for the year 2000 and projections for 2030. Diabetes Care. 2004.

[9] Rathmann W, Ward J. Socioeconomic Aspects. In: Ziegler FAGNECPALD, editor. Textbook of Diabetic Neuropathy. Stuttgart: Georg Thieme Verlag; 2003. p. 361-72.

[10] Vinik AI, Holland MT, Le Beau JM, Liuzzi FJ, Stansberry KB, Colen LB. Diabetic neuropathies. Diabetes care. 1992;15(12):1926-75. Epub 1992/12/01.

[11] Tahrani AA, Askwith T, Stevens MJ. Emerging drugs for diabetic neuropathy. Expert opinion on emerging drugs. 2010;15(4):661-83. Epub 2010/08/28.

[12] Quah JH, Luo N, Ng WY, How CH, Tay EG. Health-related quality of life is associated with diabetic complications, but not with short-term diabetic control in primary care. Annals of the Academy of Medicine, Singapore. 2011;40(6):276-86. Epub 2011/07/23.

[13] A R, Epstein S. Review of 100 cases of "diabetic neuropathy" followed from 1-10 years. The Journal of clinical endocrinology and metabolism. 1945(5):92-109.

[14] Edwards JL, Vincent AM, Cheng HT, Feldman EL. Diabetic neuropathy: mechanisms to management. Pharmacol Ther. 2008;120(1):1-34. Epub 2008/07/12.

[15] Vinik A, Mehrabyan A, Colen L, Boulton A. Focal entrapment neuropathies in diabetes. Diabetes Care. 2004;27(7):1783-8. Epub 2004/06/29.

[16] Dyck PJ, Kratz KM, Karnes JL, Litchy WJ, Klein R, Pach JM, et al. The prevalence by staged severity of various types of diabetic neuropathy, retinopathy, and nephropathy in a population-based cohort: the Rochester Diabetic Neuropathy Study. Neurology. 1993;43(4):817-24. Epub 1993/04/01.

[17] Li C, Dobrowsky RT. Targeting Molecular Chaperones in Diabetic Peripheral Neuropathy. In: Hayat G, editor. Peripheral Neuropathy - Advances in Diagnostic and Therapeutic Approaches: InTech; 2012. p. 39-62.

[18] Boulton AJ, Malik RA. Diabetic neuropathy. The Medical clinics of North America. 1998;82(4):909-29. Epub 1998/08/26.

[19] Farmer KL, Li C, Dobrowsky RT. Diabetic Peripheral Neuropathy:Should a Chaperone Accompany Our Therapeutic Approach? Pharmacol Rev. 2012. Epub 2012/08/14.

[20] Harris M, Eastman R, Cowie C. Symptoms of sensory neuropathy in adults with NIDDM in the U.S. population. Diabetes Care. 1993;16(11):1446-52. Epub 1993/11/01.

[21] Boulton AJ, Armstrong WD, Scarpello JH, Ward JD. The natural history of painful diabetic neuropathy--a 4-year study. Postgrad Med J. 1983;59(695):556-9. Epub 1983/09/01.

[22] Boulton A. Diabetic Neuropathy. Bridgewater, NJ: Aventis Pharma; 2001.

[23] Archer AG, Watkins PJ, Thomas PK, Sharma AK, Payan J. The natural history of acute painful neuropathy in diabetes mellitus. J Neurol Neurosurg Psychiatry. 1983;46(6):491-9. Epub 1983/06/01.

[24] Gooch C, Podwall D. The diabetic neuropathies. Neurologist. 2004;10(6):311-22. Epub 2004/11/03.

[25] Podwall D, Gooch C. Diabetic neuropathy: clinical features, etiology, and therapy. Curr Neurol Neurosci Rep. 2004;4(1):55-61. Epub 2003/12/20.

[26] Armstrong DG, Lavery LA, Harkless LB. Validation of a diabetic wound classification system. The contribution of depth, infection, and ischemia to risk of amputation. Diabetes Care. 1998;21(5):855-9. Epub 1998/05/20.

[27] Margolis J, Cao Z, Fowler R, Harnett J, Sanchez RJ, Mardekian J, et al. Evaluation of healthcare resource utilization and costs in employees with pain associated with dia-

betic peripheral neuropathy treated with pregabalin or duloxetine. J Med Econ. 2010;13(4):738-47. Epub 2010/11/26.

[28] Sussman C, Strauss M, Barry DD, Ayyappa E. Consideration Motor Neuropathy Neuropathic Foot. Journal of Prosthetics and Orthotics. 2005;17(2):28-31.

[29] Forsblom CM, Sane T, Groop PH, Totterman KJ, Kallio M, Saloranta C, et al. Risk factors for mortality in Type II (non-insulin-dependent) diabetes: evidence of a role for neuropathy and a protective effect of HLA-DR4. Diabetologia. 1998;41(11):1253-62. Epub 1998/12/02.

[30] Ramsey SD, Newton K, Blough D, McCulloch DK, Sandhu N, Reiber GE, et al. Incidence, outcomes, and cost of foot ulcers in patients with diabetes. Diabetes Care. 1999;22(3):382-7. Epub 1999/03/31.

[31] Coppini DV, Bowtell PA, Weng C, Young PJ, Sonksen PH. Showing neuropathy is related to increased mortality in diabetic patients - a survival analysis using an accelerated failure time model. J Clin Epidemiol. 2000;53(5):519-23. Epub 2000/05/17.

[32] DCCT. The effect of intensive diabetes therapy on the development and progression of neuropathy. The Diabetes Control and Complications Trial Research Group. Ann Intern Med. 1995;122(8):561-8. Epub 1995/04/15.

[33] DCCT. Factors in development of diabetic neuropathy. Baseline analysis of neuropathy in feasibility phase of Diabetes Control and Complications Trial (DCCT). The DCCT Research Group. Diabetes. 1988;37(4):476-81. Epub 1988/04/01.

[34] Tesfaye S, Selvarajah D. The Eurodiab study: what has this taught us about diabetic peripheral neuropathy? Curr Diab Rep. 2009;9(6):432-4. Epub 2009/12/04.

[35] Stratton IM, Adler AI, Neil HA, Matthews DR, Manley SE, Cull CA, et al. Association of glycaemia with macrovascular and microvascular complications of type 2 diabetes (UKPDS 35): prospective observational study. Bmj. 2000;321(7258):405-12. Epub 2000/08/11.

[36] Dyck PJ, Davies JL, Wilson DM, Service FJ, Melton LJ, 3rd, O'Brien PC. Risk factors for severity of diabetic polyneuropathy: intensive longitudinal assessment of the Rochester Diabetic Neuropathy Study cohort. Diabetes Care. 1999;22(9):1479-86. Epub 1999/09/10.

[37] Pirart J. [Diabetes mellitus and its degenerative complications: a prospective study of 4,400 patients observed between 1947 and 1973 (3rd and last part) (author's transl)]. Diabete Metab. 1977;3(4):245-56. Epub 1977/12/01. Diabete et complications degeneratives. Presentation d'une etude prospective portant sur 4400 cas observes entre 1947 et 1973 (troisieme et derniere partie).

[38] Pirart J. [Diabetes mellitus and its degenerative complications: a prospective study of 4,400 patients observed between 1947 and 1973 (2nd part) (author's transl)]. Diabete Metab. 1977;3(3):173-82. Epub 1977/09/01. Diabete et complications degeneratives

presentation d'une etude prospective portant sur 4400 cas observes entre 1947 et 1973 (deuxieme partie).

[39] Pirart J. [Diabetes mellitus and its degenerative complications: a prospective study of 4,400 patients observed between 1947 and 1973 (author's transl)]. Diabete Metab. 1977;3(2):97-107. Epub 1977/06/01. Diabete et complications degeneratives presentation d'une etude prospective portant sur 4400 cas observes entre 1947 et 1973. (Premiere partie).

[40] Tesfaye S, Stevens LK, Stephenson JM, Fuller JH, Plater M, Ionescu-Tirgoviste C, et al. Prevalence of diabetic peripheral neuropathy and its relation to glycaemic control and potential risk factors: the EURODIAB IDDM Complications Study. Diabetologia. 1996;39(11):1377-84. Epub 1996/11/01.

[41] Maser RE, Steenkiste AR, Dorman JS, Nielsen VK, Bass EB, Manjoo Q, et al. Epidemiological correlates of diabetic neuropathy. Report from Pittsburgh Epidemiology of Diabetes Complications Study. Diabetes. 1989;38(11):1456-61. Epub 1989/11/01.

[42] Franklin GM, Shetterly SM, Cohen JA, Baxter J, Hamman RF. Risk factors for distal symmetric neuropathy in NIDDM. The San Luis Valley Diabetes Study. Diabetes Care. 1994;17(10):1172-7. Epub 1994/10/01.

[43] Gabbay KH, Merola LO, Field RA. Sorbitol pathway: presence in nerve and cord with substrate accumulation in diabetes. Science. 1966;151(3707):209-10. Epub 1966/01/14.

[44] Hounsom L, Tomlinson DR. Does neuropathy develop in animal models? Clin Neurosci. 1997;4(6):380-9. Epub 1997/01/01.

[45] Brownlee M. Biochemistry and molecular cell biology of diabetic complications. Nature. 2001;414(6865):813-20. Epub 2001/12/14.

[46] Morrison AD, Clements RS, Jr., Travis SB, Oski F, Winegrad AI. Glucose utilization by the polyol pathway in human erythrocytes. Biochem Biophys Res Commun. 1970;40(1):199-205. Epub 1970/07/13.

[47] Kinoshita JH. A thirty year journey in the polyol pathway. Exp Eye Res. 1990;50(6): 567-73. Epub 1990/06/01.

[48] Reddy DV. Amino Acid Transport in the Lens in Relation to Sugar Cataracts. Invest Ophthalmol. 1965;4:700-8. Epub 1965/08/01.

[49] Chylack LT, Jr., Kinoshita JH. A biochemical evaluation of a cataract induced in a high-glucose medium. Invest Ophthalmol. 1969;8(4):401-12. Epub 1969/08/01.

[50] Reddy DV, Kinsey VE. Transport of amino acids into intraocular fluids and lens in diabetic rabbits. Invest Ophthalmol. 1963;2:237-42. Epub 1963/06/01.

[51] Beyer-Mears A, Cruz E. Reversal of diabetic cataract by sorbinil, an aldose reductase inhibitor. Diabetes. 1985;34(1):15-21. Epub 1985/01/01.

[52] Lee AY, Chung SK, Chung SS. Demonstration that polyol accumulation is responsible for diabetic cataract by the use of transgenic mice expressing the aldose reductase gene in the lens. Proceedings of the National Academy of Sciences of the United States of America. 1995;92(7):2780-4. Epub 1995/03/28.

[53] Tomlinson DR, Holmes PR, Mayer JH. Reversal, by treatment with an aldose reductase inhibitor, of impaired axonal transport and motor nerve conduction velocity in experimental diabetes mellitus. Neuroscience letters. 1982;31(2):189-93. Epub 1982/08/16.

[54] Obrosova IG, Pacher P, Szabo C, Zsengeller Z, Hirooka H, Stevens MJ, et al. Aldose reductase inhibition counteracts oxidative-nitrosative stress and poly(ADP-ribose) polymerase activation in tissue sites for diabetes complications. Diabetes. 2005;54(1): 234-42. Epub 2004/12/24.

[55] Gillon KR, Hawthorne JN, Tomlinson DR. Myo-inositol and sorbitol metabolism in relation to peripheral nerve function in experimental diabetes in the rat: the effect of aldose reductase inhibition. Diabetologia. 1983;25(4):365-71. Epub 1983/10/01.

[56] Drel VR, Mashtalir N, Ilnytska O, Shin J, Li F, Lyzogubov VV, et al. The leptin-deficient (ob/ob) mouse: a new animal model of peripheral neuropathy of type 2 diabetes and obesity. Diabetes. 2006;55(12):3335-43. Epub 2006/11/30.

[57] Stewart MA, Sherman WR, Anthony S. Free sugars in alloxan diabetic rat nerve. Biochem Biophys Res Commun. 1966;22(5):4-91. Epub 1966/03/08.

[58] Yagihashi S, Kamijo M, Ido Y, Mirrlees DJ. Effects of long-term aldose reductase inhibition on development of experimental diabetic neuropathy. Ultrastructural and morphometric studies of sural nerve in streptozocin-induced diabetic rats. Diabetes. 1990;39(6):690-6. Epub 1990/06/01.

[59] Kato N, Mizuno K, Makino M, Suzuki T, Yagihashi S. Effects of 15-month aldose reductase inhibition with fidarestat on the experimental diabetic neuropathy in rats. Diabetes Res Clin Pract. 2000;50(2):77-85. Epub 2000/08/29.

[60] Sima AA, Prashar A, Zhang WX, Chakrabarti S, Greene DA. Preventive effect of long-term aldose reductase inhibition (ponalrestat) on nerve conduction and sural nerve structure in the spontaneously diabetic Bio-Breeding rat. J Clin Invest. 1990;85(5):1410-20. Epub 1990/05/01.

[61] Yagihashi S, Yamagishi SI, Wada Ri R, Baba M, Hohman TC, Yabe-Nishimura C, et al. Neuropathy in diabetic mice overexpressing human aldose reductase and effects of aldose reductase inhibitor. Brain : a journal of neurology. 2001;124(Pt 12):2448-58. Epub 2001/11/10.

[62] Song Z, Fu DT, Chan YS, Leung S, Chung SS, Chung SK. Transgenic mice overexpressing aldose reductase in Schwann cells show more severe nerve conduction ve-

locity deficit and oxidative stress under hyperglycemic stress. Molecular and cellular neurosciences. 2003;23(4):638-47. Epub 2003/08/23.

[63] Ho EC, Lam KS, Chen YS, Yip JC, Arvindakshan M, Yamagishi S, et al. Aldose reductase-deficient mice are protected from delayed motor nerve conduction velocity, increased c-Jun NH2-terminal kinase activation, depletion of reduced glutathione, increased superoxide accumulation, and DNA damage. Diabetes. 2006;55(7):1946-53. Epub 2006/06/29.

[64] Hayman S, Kinoshita JH. Isolation and Properties of Lens Aldose Reductase. The Journal of biological chemistry. 1965;240:877-82. Epub 1965/02/01.

[65] Mizisin AP, Kalichman MW, Bache M, Dines KC, DiStefano PS. NT-3 attenuates functional and structural disorders in sensory nerves of galactose-fed rats. Journal of neuropathology and experimental neurology. 1998;57(9):803-13. Epub 1998/09/16.

[66] Gabbay KH, JJ. S. Nerve conduction defect in galactose-fed rats. Diabetes. 1972(21): 295-300.

[67] Calcutt NA, Tomlinson DR, Biswas S. Coexistence of nerve conduction deficit with increased Na(+)-K(+)-ATPase activity in galactose-fed mice. Implications for polyol pathway and diabetic neuropathy. Diabetes. 1990;39(6):663-6. Epub 1990/06/01.

[68] Levy HL, Hammersen G. Newborn screening for galactosemia and other galactose metabolic defects. The Journal of pediatrics. 1978;92(6):871-7. Epub 1978/06/01.

[69] Lambourne JE, Tomlinson DR, Brown AM, Willars GB. Opposite effects of diabetes and galactosaemia on adenosine triphosphatase activity in rat nervous tissue. Diabetologia. 1987;30(5):360-2. Epub 1987/05/01.

[70] Kalichman MW, Dines KC, Bobik M, Mizisin AP. Nerve conduction velocity, laser Doppler flow, and axonal caliber in galactose and streptozotocin diabetes. Brain research. 1998;810(1-2):130-7. Epub 1998/11/14.

[71] Engerman RL, Kern TS, Larson ME. Nerve conduction velocity in dogs is reduced by diabetes and not by galactosemia. Metabolism: clinical and experimental. 1990;39(6): 638-40. Epub 1990/06/01.

[72] Clements RS, Jr. The polyol pathway. A historical review. Drugs. 1986;32 Suppl 2:3-5. Epub 1986/01/01.

[73] Oates PJ. Polyol pathway and diabetic peripheral neuropathy. Int Rev Neurobiol. 2002;50:325-92. Epub 2002/08/30.

[74] Rivelli JF, Amaiden MR, Monesterolo NE, Previtali G, Santander VS, Fernandez A, et al. High glucose levels induce inhibition of Na,K-ATPase via stimulation of aldose reductase, formation of microtubules and formation of an acetylated tubulin/Na,K-ATPase complex. Int J Biochem Cell Biol. 2012;44(8):1203-13. Epub 2012/05/09.

[75] Duby JJ, Campbell RK, Setter SM, White JR, Rasmussen KA. Diabetic neuropathy: an intensive review. Am J Health Syst Pharm. 2004;61(2):160-73; quiz 75-6. Epub 2004/01/31.

[76] Lee AY, Chung SS. Contributions of polyol pathway to oxidative stress in diabetic cataract. FASEB journal : official publication of the Federation of American Societies for Experimental Biology. 1999;13(1):23-30. Epub 1999/01/05.

[77] Yabe-Nishimura C. Aldose reductase in glucose toxicity: a potential target for the prevention of diabetic complications. Pharmacol Rev. 1998;50(1):21-33. Epub 1998/04/29.

[78] Hale PJ, Nattrass M, Silverman SH, Sennit C, Perkins CM, Uden A, et al. Peripheral nerve concentrations of glucose, fructose, sorbitol and myoinositol in diabetic and non-diabetic patients. Diabetologia. 1987;30(7):464-7. Epub 1987/07/01.

[79] Dyck PJ, Sherman WR, Hallcher LM, Service FJ, O'Brien PC, Grina LA, et al. Human diabetic endoneurial sorbitol, fructose, and myo-inositol related to sural nerve morphometry. Ann Neurol. 1980;8(6):590-6. Epub 1980/12/01.

[80] Dyck PJ, Zimmerman BR, Vilen TH, Minnerath SR, Karnes JL, Yao JK, et al. Nerve glucose, fructose, sorbitol, myo-inositol, and fiber degeneration and regeneration in diabetic neuropathy. N Engl J Med. 1988;319(9):542-8. Epub 1988/09/01.

[81] Sima AA, Dunlap JA, Davidson EP, Wiese TJ, Lightle RL, Greene DA, et al. Supplemental myo-inositol prevents L-fucose-induced diabetic neuropathy. Diabetes. 1997;46(2):301-6. Epub 1997/02/01.

[82] Mayer JH, Tomlinson DR. Prevention of defects of axonal transport and nerve conduction velocity by oral administration of myo-inositol or an aldose reductase inhibitor in streptozotocin-diabetic rats. Diabetologia. 1983;25(5):433-8. Epub 1983/11/01.

[83] Gregersen G, Bertelsen B, Harbo H, Larsen E, Andersen JR, Helles A, et al. Oral supplementation of myoinositol: effects on peripheral nerve function in human diabetics and on the concentration in plasma, erythrocytes, urine and muscle tissue in human diabetics and normals. Acta Neurol Scand. 1983;67(3):164-72. Epub 1983/03/01.

[84] Gregersen G, Borsting H, Theil P, Servo C. Myoinositol and function of peripheral nerves in human diabetics. A controlled clinical trial. Acta Neurol Scand. 1978;58(4): 241-8. Epub 1978/10/01.

[85] Fukushi S, Merola LO, Kinoshita JH. Altering the course of cataracts in diabetic rats. Invest Ophthalmol Vis Sci. 1980;19(3):313-5. Epub 1980/03/01.

[86] Ashizawa N, Yoshida M, Sugiyama Y, Akaike N, Ohbayashi S, Aotsuka T, et al. Effects of a novel potent aldose reductase inhibitor, GP-1447, on aldose reductase activity in vitro and on diabetic neuropathy and cataract formation in rats. Jpn J Pharmacol. 1997;73(2):133-44. Epub 1997/02/01.

[87] Yagihashi S, Yamagishi SI, Wada Ri R, Baba M, Hohman TC, Yabe-Nishimura C, et al. Neuropathy in diabetic mice overexpressing human aldose reductase and effects of aldose reductase inhibitor. Brain. 2001;124(Pt 12):2448-58. Epub 2001/11/10.

[88] Cameron NE, Cotter MA, Robertson S. The effect of aldose reductase inhibition on the pattern of nerve conduction deficits in diabetic rats. Q J Exp Physiol. 1989;74(6): 917-26. Epub 1989/11/01.

[89] Calcutt NA, Freshwater JD, Mizisin AP. Prevention of sensory disorders in diabetic Sprague-Dawley rats by aldose reductase inhibition or treatment with ciliary neurotrophic factor. Diabetologia. 2004;47(4):718-24. Epub 2004/08/10.

[90] Yang B, Millward A, Demaine A. Functional differences between the susceptibility Z-2/C-106 and protective Z+2/T-106 promoter region polymorphisms of the aldose reductase gene may account for the association with diabetic microvascular complications. Biochim Biophys Acta. 2003;1639(1):1-7. Epub 2003/08/29.

[91] Demaine AG. Polymorphisms of the aldose reductase gene and susceptibility to diabetic microvascular complications. Curr Med Chem. 2003;10(15):1389-98. Epub 2003/07/23.

[92] Donaghue KC, Margan SH, Chan AK, Holloway B, Silink M, Rangel T, et al. The association of aldose reductase gene (AKR1B1) polymorphisms with diabetic neuropathy in adolescents. Diabet Med. 2005;22(10):1315-20. Epub 2005/09/24.

[93] Thamotharampillai K, Chan AK, Bennetts B, Craig ME, Cusumano J, Silink M, et al. Decline in neurophysiological function after 7 years in an adolescent diabetic cohort and the role of aldose reductase gene polymorphisms. Diabetes Care. 2006;29(9): 2053-7. Epub 2006/08/29.

[94] Pollreisz A, Schmidt-Erfurth U. Diabetic cataract-pathogenesis, epidemiology and treatment. J Ophthalmol. 2010;2010:608751. Epub 2010/07/17.

[95] Bron AJ, Sparrow J, Brown NA, Harding JJ, Blakytny R. The lens in diabetes. Eye (Lond). 1993;7 (Pt 2):260-75. Epub 1993/01/01.

[96] Handelsman DJ, Turtle JR. Clinical trial of an aldose reductase inhibitor in diabetic neuropathy. Diabetes. 1981;30(6):459-64. Epub 1981/06/01.

[97] Gabbay KH, Spack N, Loo S, Hirsch HJ, Ackil AA. Aldose reductase inhibition: studies with alrestatin. Metabolism. 1979;28(4 Suppl 1):471-6. Epub 1979/04/01.

[98] Sima AA, Bril V, Nathaniel V, McEwen TA, Brown MB, Lattimer SA, et al. Regeneration and repair of myelinated fibers in sural-nerve biopsy specimens from patients with diabetic neuropathy treated with sorbinil. N Engl J Med. 1988;319(9):548-55. Epub 1988/09/01.

[99] Judzewitsch RG, Jaspan JB, Polonsky KS, Weinberg CR, Halter JB, Halar E, et al. Aldose reductase inhibition improves nerve conduction velocity in diabetic patients. N Engl J Med. 1983;308(3):119-25. Epub 1983/01/20.

[100] Young RJ, Ewing DJ, Clarke BF. A controlled trial of sorbinil, an aldose reductase inhibitor, in chronic painful diabetic neuropathy. Diabetes. 1983;32(10):938-42. Epub 1983/10/01.

[101] Lewin IG, O'Brien IA, Morgan MH, Corrall RJ. Clinical and neurophysiological studies with the aldose reductase inhibitor, sorbinil, in symptomatic diabetic neuropathy. Diabetologia. 1984;26(6):445-8. Epub 1984/06/01.

[102] Sundkvist G, Lilja B, Rosen I, Agardh CD. Autonomic and peripheral nerve function in early diabetic neuropathy. Possible influence of a novel aldose reductase inhibitor on autonomic function. Acta Med Scand. 1987;221(5):445-53. Epub 1987/01/01.

[103] Giugliano D, Marfella R, Quatraro A, De Rosa N, Salvatore T, Cozzolino D, et al. Tolrestat for mild diabetic neuropathy. A 52-week, randomized, placebo-controlled trial. Ann Intern Med. 1993;118(1):7-11. Epub 1993/01/01.

[104] Giugliano D, Acampora R, Marfella R, Di Maro G, De Rosa N, Misso L, et al. Tolrestat in the primary prevention of diabetic neuropathy. Diabetes Care. 1995;18(4): 536-41. Epub 1995/04/01.

[105] Nicolucci A, Carinci F, Graepel JG, Hohman TC, Ferris F, Lachin JM. The efficacy of tolrestat in the treatment of diabetic peripheral neuropathy. A meta-analysis of individual patient data. Diabetes Care. 1996;19(10):1091-6. Epub 1996/10/01.

[106] Boulton AJ, Levin S, Comstock J. A multicentre trial of the aldose-reductase inhibitor, tolrestat, in patients with symptomatic diabetic neuropathy. Diabetologia. 1990;33(7): 431-7. Epub 1990/07/01.

[107] Aronson JK. Aldose Reductase Inhibitors. Meyler's Side Effects of Endocrine and Metabolic Drugs. San Diego: Elservier; 2009. p. 359.

[108] Greene DA, Sima AA. Effects of aldose reductase inhibitors on the progression of nerve damage. Diabet Med. 1993;10 Suppl 2:31S-2S. Epub 1993/01/01.

[109] Stribling D, Mirrlees DJ, Harrison HE, Earl DC. Properties of ICI 128,436, a novel aldose reductase inhibitor, and its effects on diabetic complications in the rat. Metabolism. 1985;34(4):336-44. Epub 1985/04/01.

[110] Krentz AJ, Honigsberger L, Ellis SH, Hardman M, Nattrass M. A 12-month randomized controlled study of the aldose reductase inhibitor ponalrestat in patients with chronic symptomatic diabetic neuropathy. Diabet Med. 1992;9(5):463-8. Epub 1992/06/01.

[111] Arezzo J, Klioze S, Peterson M, Lakshminarayanan M. Zopolrestat phase II neuropathy study group: efficacy and safety results of a phase II multicenter study of the al-

dose reductase inhibitor zopolrestat in patients with peripheral symmetrical diabetic polyneuropathy. Diabetes Care. 1996;45(2):276A.

[112] Greene DA, Arezzo JC, Brown MB. Effect of aldose reductase inhibition on nerve conduction and morphometry in diabetic neuropathy. Zenarestat Study Group. Neurology. 1999;53(3):580-91. Epub 1999/08/17.

[113] Bril V, Buchanan RA. Long-term effects of ranirestat (AS-3201) on peripheral nerve function in patients with diabetic sensorimotor polyneuropathy. Diabetes Care. 2006;29(1):68-72. Epub 2005/12/24.

[114] Bril V, Hirose T, Tomioka S, Buchanan R. Ranirestat for the management of diabetic sensorimotor polyneuropathy. Diabetes Care. 2009;32(7):1256-60. Epub 2009/04/16.

[115] Hotta N, Toyota T, Matsuoka K, Shigeta Y, Kikkawa R, Kaneko T, et al. Clinical efficacy of fidarestat, a novel aldose reductase inhibitor, for diabetic peripheral neuropathy: a 52-week multicenter placebo-controlled double-blind parallel group study. Diabetes Care. 2001;24(10):1776-82. Epub 2001/09/28.

[116] Giannoukakis N. Fidarestat. Sanwa Kagaku/NC Curex/Sankyo. Curr Opin Investig Drugs. 2003;4(10):1233-9. Epub 2003/12/03.

[117] Hotta N, Akanuma Y, Kawamori R, Matsuoka K, Oka Y, Shichiri M, et al. Long-term clinical effects of epalrestat, an aldose reductase inhibitor, on diabetic peripheral neuropathy: the 3-year, multicenter, comparative Aldose Reductase Inhibitor-Diabetes Complications Trial. Diabetes Care. 2006;29(7):1538-44. Epub 2006/06/28.

[118] Gabbay KH. Aldose reductase inhibition in the treatment of diabetic neuropathy: where are we in 2004? Curr Diab Rep. 2004;4(6):405-8. Epub 2004/11/13.

[119] Chalk C, Benstead TJ, Moore F. Aldose reductase inhibitors for the treatment of diabetic polyneuropathy. Cochrane Database Syst Rev. 2007(4):CD004572. Epub 2007/10/19.

[120] Airey M, Bennett C, Nicolucci A, Williams R. Aldose reductase inhibitors for the prevention and treatment of diabetic peripheral neuropathy. Cochrane Database Syst Rev. 2000(2):CD002182. Epub 2000/05/05.

[121] Thornalley PJ, Langborg A, Minhas HS. Formation of glyoxal, methylglyoxal and 3-deoxyglucosone in the glycation of proteins by glucose. Biochem J. 1999;344 Pt 1:109-16. Epub 1999/11/05.

[122] Thornalley PJ. Glycation in diabetic neuropathy: characteristics, consequences, causes, and therapeutic options. Int Rev Neurobiol. 2002;50:37-57. Epub 2002/08/30.

[123] Giardino I, Edelstein D, Brownlee M. Nonenzymatic glycosylation in vitro and in bovine endothelial cells alters basic fibroblast growth factor activity. A model for intracellular glycosylation in diabetes. J Clin Invest. 1994;94(1):110-7. Epub 1994/07/01.

[124] Shinohara M, Thornalley PJ, Giardino I, Beisswenger P, Thorpe SR, Onorato J, et al. Overexpression of glyoxalase-I in bovine endothelial cells inhibits intracellular ad-

vanced glycation endproduct formation and prevents hyperglycemia-induced increases in macromolecular endocytosis. J Clin Invest. 1998;101(5):1142-7. Epub 1998/04/16.

[125] McLean WG, Pekiner C, Cullum NA, Casson IF. Posttranslational modifications of nerve cytoskeletal proteins in experimental diabetes. Mol Neurobiol. 1992;6(2-3): 225-37. Epub 1992/01/01.

[126] Williams SK, Howarth NL, Devenny JJ, Bitensky MW. Structural and functional consequences of increased tubulin glycosylation in diabetes mellitus. Proc Natl Acad Sci U S A. 1982;79(21):6546-50. Epub 1982/11/01.

[127] Huijberts MS, Wolffenbuttel BH, Boudier HA, Crijns FR, Kruseman AC, Poitevin P, et al. Aminoguanidine treatment increases elasticity and decreases fluid filtration of large arteries from diabetic rats. J Clin Invest. 1993;92(3):1407-11. Epub 1993/09/01.

[128] Soulis-Liparota T, Cooper M, Papazoglou D, Clarke B, Jerums G. Retardation by aminoguanidine of development of albuminuria, mesangial expansion, and tissue fluorescence in streptozocin-induced diabetic rat. Diabetes. 1991;40(10):1328-34. Epub 1991/10/01.

[129] Sensi M, Morano S, Morelli S, Castaldo P, Sagratella E, De Rossi MG, et al. Reduction of advanced glycation end-product (AGE) levels in nervous tissue proteins of diabetic Lewis rats following islet transplants is related to different durations of poor metabolic control. Eur J Neurosci. 1998;10(9):2768-75. Epub 1998/10/03.

[130] Ryle C, Donaghy M. Non-enzymatic glycation of peripheral nerve proteins in human diabetics. J Neurol Sci. 1995;129(1):62-8. Epub 1995/03/01.

[131] Ryle C, Leow CK, Donaghy M. Nonenzymatic glycation of peripheral and central nervous system proteins in experimental diabetes mellitus. Muscle Nerve. 1997;20(5): 577-84. Epub 1997/05/01.

[132] Edelstein D, Brownlee M. Mechanistic studies of advanced glycosylation end product inhibition by aminoguanidine. Diabetes. 1992;41(1):26-9. Epub 1992/01/01.

[133] Tilton RG, Chang K, Hasan KS, Smith SR, Petrash JM, Misko TP, et al. Prevention of diabetic vascular dysfunction by guanidines. Inhibition of nitric oxide synthase versus advanced glycation end-product formation. Diabetes. 1993;42(2):221-32. Epub 1993/02/01.

[134] Yu PH, Zuo DM. Aminoguanidine inhibits semicarbazide-sensitive amine oxidase activity: implications for advanced glycation and diabetic complications. Diabetologia. 1997;40(11):1243-50. Epub 1997/12/06.

[135] Giardino I, Fard AK, Hatchell DL, Brownlee M. Aminoguanidine inhibits reactive oxygen species formation, lipid peroxidation, and oxidant-induced apoptosis. Diabetes. 1998;47(7):1114-20. Epub 1998/07/02.

[136] Soulis T, Cooper ME, Vranes D, Bucala R, Jerums G. Effects of aminoguanidine in preventing experimental diabetic nephropathy are related to the duration of treatment. Kidney Int. 1996;50(2):627-34. Epub 1996/08/01.

[137] Miyauchi Y, Shikama H, Takasu T, Okamiya H, Umeda M, Hirasaki E, et al. Slowing of peripheral motor nerve conduction was ameliorated by aminoguanidine in streptozocin-induced diabetic rats. Eur J Endocrinol. 1996;134(4):467-73. Epub 1996/04/01.

[138] Sugimoto K, Yagihashi S. Effects of aminoguanidine on structural alterations of microvessels in peripheral nerve of streptozotocin diabetic rats. Microvasc Res. 1997;53(2):105-12. Epub 1997/03/01.

[139] Kihara M, Schmelzer JD, Poduslo JF, Curran GL, Nickander KK, Low PA. Aminoguanidine effects on nerve blood flow, vascular permeability, electrophysiology, and oxygen free radicals. Proc Natl Acad Sci U S A. 1991;88(14):6107-11. Epub 1991/07/15.

[140] Cameron NE, Cotter MA, Dines K, Love A. Effects of aminoguanidine on peripheral nerve function and polyol pathway metabolites in streptozotocin-diabetic rats. Diabetologia. 1992;35(10):946-50. Epub 1992/10/01.

[141] Duran-Jimenez B, Dobler D, Moffatt S, Rabbani N, Streuli CH, Thornalley PJ, et al. Advanced glycation end products in extracellular matrix proteins contribute to the failure of sensory nerve regeneration in diabetes. Diabetes. 2009;58(12):2893-903. Epub 2009/09/02.

[142] Birrell AM, Heffernan SJ, Ansselin AD, McLennan S, Church DK, Gillin AG, et al. Functional and structural abnormalities in the nerves of type I diabetic baboons: aminoguanidine treatment does not improve nerve function. Diabetologia. 2000;43(1): 110-6. Epub 2000/02/15.

[143] Freedman BI, Wuerth JP, Cartwright K, Bain RP, Dippe S, Hershon K, et al. Design and baseline characteristics for the aminoguanidine Clinical Trial in Overt Type 2 Diabetic Nephropathy (ACTION II). Control Clin Trials. 1999;20(5):493-510. Epub 1999/09/30.

[144] Bolton WK, Cattran DC, Williams ME, Adler SG, Appel GB, Cartwright K, et al. Randomized trial of an inhibitor of formation of advanced glycation end products in diabetic nephropathy. Am J Nephrol. 2004;24(1):32-40. Epub 2003/12/20.

[145] Das Evcimen N, King GL. The role of protein kinase C activation and the vascular complications of diabetes. Pharmacol Res. 2007;55(6):498-510. Epub 2007/06/19.

[146] Eichberg J. Protein kinase C changes in diabetes: is the concept relevant to neuropathy? Int Rev Neurobiol. 2002;50:61-82. Epub 2002/08/30.

[147] Kim J, Rushovich EH, Thomas TP, Ueda T, Agranoff BW, Greene DA. Diminished specific activity of cytosolic protein kinase C in sciatic nerve of streptozocin-induced diabetic rats and its correction by dietary myo-inositol. Diabetes. 1991;40(11):1545-54. Epub 1991/11/01.

[148] Cameron NE, Cotter MA, Jack AM, Basso MD, Hohman TC. Protein kinase C effects on nerve function, perfusion, Na(+), K(+)-ATPase activity and glutathione content in diabetic rats. Diabetologia. 1999;42(9):1120-30. Epub 1999/08/14.

[149] Xia P, Kramer RM, King GL. Identification of the mechanism for the inhibition of Na +,K(+)-adenosine triphosphatase by hyperglycemia involving activation of protein kinase C and cytosolic phospholipase A2. J Clin Invest. 1995;96(2):733-40. Epub 1995/08/01.

[150] Nakamura J, Kato K, Hamada Y, Nakayama M, Chaya S, Nakashima E, et al. A protein kinase C-beta-selective inhibitor ameliorates neural dysfunction in streptozotocin-induced diabetic rats. Diabetes. 1999;48(10):2090-5. Epub 1999/10/08.

[151] Cameron NE, Cotter MA. Effects of protein kinase Cbeta inhibition on neurovascular dysfunction in diabetic rats: interaction with oxidative stress and essential fatty acid dysmetabolism. Diabetes Metab Res Rev. 2002;18(4):315-23. Epub 2002/08/31.

[152] Casellini CM, Barlow PM, Rice AL, Casey M, Simmons K, Pittenger G, et al. A 6-month, randomized, double-masked, placebo-controlled study evaluating the effects of the protein kinase C-beta inhibitor ruboxistaurin on skin microvascular blood flow and other measures of diabetic peripheral neuropathy. Diabetes Care. 2007;30(4): 896-902. Epub 2007/03/30.

[153] Boyd A, Casselini C, Vinik E, Vinik A. Quality of life and objective measures of diabetic neuropathy in a prospective placebo-controlled trial of ruboxistaurin and topiramate. J Diabetes Sci Technol. 2011;5(3):714-22. Epub 2011/07/05.

[154] Vinik AI, Bril V, Kempler P, Litchy WJ, Tesfaye S, Price KL, et al. Treatment of symptomatic diabetic peripheral neuropathy with the protein kinase C beta-inhibitor ruboxistaurin mesylate during a 1-year, randomized, placebo-controlled, double-blind clinical trial. Clin Ther. 2005;27(8):1164-80. Epub 2005/10/04.

[155] Apfel SC. Nerve growth factor for the treatment of diabetic neuropathy: what went wrong, what went right, and what does the future hold? Int Rev Neurobiol. 2002;50:393-413. Epub 2002/08/30.

[156] Leinninger GM, Vincent AM, Feldman EL. The role of growth factors in diabetic peripheral neuropathy. J Peripher Nerv Syst. 2004;9(1):26-53. Epub 2004/02/12.

[157] Kasayama S, Oka T. Impaired production of nerve growth factor in the submandibular gland of diabetic mice. Am J Physiol. 1989;257(3 Pt 1):E400-4. Epub 1989/09/01.

[158] Hellweg R, Hartung HD. Endogenous levels of nerve growth factor (NGF) are altered in experimental diabetes mellitus: a possible role for NGF in the pathogenesis of diabetic neuropathy. J Neurosci Res. 1990;26(2):258-67. Epub 1990/06/01.

[159] Fernyhough P, Diemel LT, Brewster WJ, Tomlinson DR. Deficits in sciatic nerve neuropeptide content coincide with a reduction in target tissue nerve growth factor mes-

senger RNA in streptozotocin-diabetic rats: effects of insulin treatment. Neuroscience. 1994;62(2):337-44. Epub 1994/09/01.

[160] Fernyhough P, Diemel LT, Brewster WJ, Tomlinson DR. Altered neurotrophin mRNA levels in peripheral nerve and skeletal muscle of experimentally diabetic rats. J Neurochem. 1995;64(3):1231-7. Epub 1995/03/01.

[161] Fernyhough P, Diemel LT, Tomlinson DR. Target tissue production and axonal transport of neurotrophin-3 are reduced in streptozotocin-diabetic rats. Diabetologia. 1998;41(3):300-6. Epub 1998/04/16.

[162] Rodriguez-Pena A, Botana M, Gonzalez M, Requejo F. Expression of neurotrophins and their receptors in sciatic nerve of experimentally diabetic rats. Neurosci Lett. 1995;200(1):37-40. Epub 1995/11/10.

[163] Cai F, Tomlinson DR, Fernyhough P. Elevated expression of neurotrophin-3 mRNA in sensory nerve of streptozotocin-diabetic rats. Neurosci Lett. 1999;263(2-3):81-4. Epub 1999/04/23.

[164] Mizisin AP, DiStefano PS, Liu X, Garrett DN, Tonra JR. Decreased accumulation of endogenous brain-derived neurotrophic factor against constricting sciatic nerve ligatures in streptozotocin-diabetic and galactose-fed rats. Neurosci Lett. 1999;263(2-3):149-52. Epub 1999/04/23.

[165] Hellweg R, Raivich G, Hartung HD, Hock C, Kreutzberg GW. Axonal transport of endogenous nerve growth factor (NGF) and NGF receptor in experimental diabetic neuropathy. Exp Neurol. 1994;130(1):24-30. Epub 1994/11/01.

[166] Ekstrom AR, Kanje M, Skottner A. Nerve regeneration and serum levels of insulin-like growth factor-I in rats with streptozotocin-induced insulin deficiency. Brain Res. 1989;496(1-2):141-7. Epub 1989/09/04.

[167] Wuarin L, Guertin DM, Ishii DN. Early reduction in insulin-like growth factor gene expression in diabetic nerve. Exp Neurol. 1994;130(1):106-14. Epub 1994/11/01.

[168] Calcutt NA, Muir D, Powell HC, Mizisin AP. Reduced ciliary neuronotrophic factor-like activity in nerves from diabetic or galactose-fed rats. Brain Res. 1992;575(2):320-4. Epub 1992/03/20.

[169] Xu G, Sima AA. Altered immediate early gene expression in injured diabetic nerve: implications in regeneration. J Neuropathol Exp Neurol. 2001;60(10):972-83. Epub 2001/10/09.

[170] Mizisin AP, Vu Y, Shuff M, Calcutt NA. Ciliary neurotrophic factor improves nerve conduction and ameliorates regeneration deficits in diabetic rats. Diabetes. 2004;53(7):1807-12. Epub 2004/06/29.

[171] Faradji V, Sotelo J. Low serum levels of nerve growth factor in diabetic neuropathy. Acta Neurol Scand. 1990;81(5):402-6. Epub 1990/05/01.

[172] Kim HC, Cho YJ, Ahn CW, Park KS, Kim JC, Nam JS, et al. Nerve growth factor and expression of its receptors in patients with diabetic neuropathy. Diabet Med. 2009;26(12):1228-34. Epub 2009/12/17.

[173] Anand P, Terenghi G, Warner G, Kopelman P, Williams-Chestnut RE, Sinicropi DV. The role of endogenous nerve growth factor in human diabetic neuropathy. Nat Med. 1996;2(6):703-7. Epub 1996/06/01.

[174] Diemel LT, Cai F, Anand P, Warner G, Kopelman PG, Fernyhough P, et al. Increased nerve growth factor mRNA in lateral calf skin biopsies from diabetic patients. Diabet Med. 1999;16(2):113-8. Epub 1999/05/06.

[175] Kennedy AJ, Wellmer A, Facer P, Saldanha G, Kopelman P, Lindsay RM, et al. Neurotrophin-3 is increased in skin in human diabetic neuropathy. J Neurol Neurosurg Psychiatry. 1998;65(3):393-5. Epub 1998/09/05.

[176] Lee DA, Gross L, Wittrock DA, Windebank AJ. Localization and expression of ciliary neurotrophic factor (CNTF) in postmortem sciatic nerve from patients with motor neuron disease and diabetic neuropathy. J Neuropathol Exp Neurol. 1996;55(8): 915-23. Epub 1996/08/01.

[177] Grandis M, Nobbio L, Abbruzzese M, Banchi L, Minuto F, Barreca A, et al. Insulin treatment enhances expression of IGF-I in sural nerves of diabetic patients. Muscle Nerve. 2001;24(5):622-9. Epub 2001/04/24.

[178] Kamiya H, Zhang W, Ekberg K, Wahren J, Sima AA. C-Peptide reverses nociceptive neuropathy in type 1 diabetes. Diabetes. 2006;55(12):3581-7. Epub 2006/11/30.

[179] Terenghi G, Mann D, Kopelman PG, Anand P. trkA and trkC expression is increased in human diabetic skin. Neurosci Lett. 1997;228(1):33-6. Epub 1997/05/30.

[180] Apfel SC, Kessler JA, Adornato BT, Litchy WJ, Sanders C, Rask CA. Recombinant human nerve growth factor in the treatment of diabetic polyneuropathy. NGF Study Group. Neurology. 1998;51(3):695-702. Epub 1998/09/25.

[181] Apfel SC, Schwartz S, Adornato BT, Freeman R, Biton V, Rendell M, et al. Efficacy and safety of recombinant human nerve growth factor in patients with diabetic polyneuropathy: A randomized controlled trial. rhNGF Clinical Investigator Group. Jama. 2000;284(17):2215-21. Epub 2000/11/01.

[182] Jubran M, Widenfalk J. Repair of peripheral nerve transections with fibrin sealant containing neurotrophic factors. Exp Neurol. 2003;181(2):204-12. Epub 2003/06/05.

[183] Ma QP, Woolf CJ. The progressive tactile hyperalgesia induced by peripheral inflammation is nerve growth factor dependent. Neuroreport. 1997;8(4):807-10. Epub 1997/03/03.

[184] Mills CD, Nguyen T, Tanga FY, Zhong C, Gauvin DM, Mikusa J, et al. Characterization of nerve growth factor-induced mechanical and thermal hypersensitivity in rats. Eur J Pain. 2012. Epub 2012/08/24.

[185] Weinkauf B, Obreja O, Schmelz M, Rukwied R. Differential effects of lidocaine on nerve growth factor (NGF)-evoked heat- and mechanical hyperalgesia in humans. Eur J Pain. 2012;16(4):543-9. Epub 2012/03/08.

[186] Zahn PK, Subieta A, Park SS, Brennan TJ. Effect of blockade of nerve growth factor and tumor necrosis factor on pain behaviors after plantar incision. J Pain. 2004;5(3): 157-63. Epub 2004/04/24.

[187] Halvorson KG, Kubota K, Sevcik MA, Lindsay TH, Sotillo JE, Ghilardi JR, et al. A blocking antibody to nerve growth factor attenuates skeletal pain induced by prostate tumor cells growing in bone. Cancer Res. 2005;65(20):9426-35. Epub 2005/10/19.

[188] Shelton DL, Zeller J, Ho WH, Pons J, Rosenthal A. Nerve growth factor mediates hyperalgesia and cachexia in auto-immune arthritis. Pain. 2005;116(1-2):8-16. Epub 2005/06/02.

[189] Brown MT, Murphy FT, Radin DM, Davignon I, Smith MD, West CR. Tanezumab Reduces Osteoarthritic Knee Pain: Results of a Randomized, Double-Blind, Placebo-Controlled Phase III Trial. J Pain. 2012;13(8):790-8. Epub 2012/07/13.

[190] Wellmer A, Misra VP, Sharief MK, Kopelman PG, Anand P. A double-blind placebo-controlled clinical trial of recombinant human brain-derived neurotrophic factor (rhBDNF) in diabetic polyneuropathy. J Peripher Nerv Syst. 2001;6(4):204-10. Epub 2002/01/22.

[191] Russo VC, Gluckman PD, Feldman EL, Werther GA. The insulin-like growth factor system and its pleiotropic functions in brain. Endocr Rev. 2005;26(7):916-43. Epub 2005/09/01.

[192] Bongioanni P, Reali C, Sogos V. Ciliary neurotrophic factor (CNTF) for amyotrophic lateral sclerosis/motor neuron disease. Cochrane Database Syst Rev. 2004(3):CD004302. Epub 2004/07/22.

[193] Gregory JA, Jolivalt CG, Goor J, Mizisin AP, Calcutt NA. Hypertension-induced peripheral neuropathy and the combined effects of hypertension and diabetes on nerve structure and function in rats. Acta Neuropathol. 2012;124(4):561-73. Epub 2012/07/14.

[194] Hogikyan RV, Wald JJ, Feldman EL, Greene DA, Halter JB, Supiano MA. Acute effects of adrenergic-mediated ischemia on nerve conduction in subjects with type 2 diabetes. Metabolism. 1999;48(4):495-500. Epub 1999/04/17.

[195] Cameron NE, Cotter MA, Ferguson K, Robertson S, Radcliffe MA. Effects of chronic alpha-adrenergic receptor blockade on peripheral nerve conduction, hypoxic resist-

ance, polyols, Na(+)-K(+)-ATPase activity, and vascular supply in STZ-D rats. Diabetes. 1991;40(12):1652-8. Epub 1991/12/01.

[196] Robertson S, Cameron NE, Cotter MA. The effect of the calcium antagonist nifedipine on peripheral nerve function in streptozotocin-diabetic rats. Diabetologia. 1992;35(12):1113-7. Epub 1992/12/01.

[197] Hotta N, Kakuta H, Fukasawa H, Koh N, Sakakibara F, Komori H, et al. Effect of niceritrol on streptozocin-induced diabetic neuropathy in rats. Diabetes. 1992;41(5): 587-91. Epub 1992/05/01.

[198] Malik RA, Tomlinson DR. Angiotensin-converting enzyme inhibitors: are there credible mechanisms for beneficial effects in diabetic neuropathy? Int Rev Neurobiol. 2002;50:415-30. Epub 2002/08/30.

[199] Coppey LJ, Davidson EP, Rinehart TW, Gellett JS, Oltman CL, Lund DD, et al. ACE inhibitor or angiotensin II receptor antagonist attenuates diabetic neuropathy in streptozotocin-induced diabetic rats. Diabetes. 2006;55(2):341-8. Epub 2006/01/31.

[200] Cameron NE, Cotter MA, Robertson S. Angiotensin converting enzyme inhibition prevents development of muscle and nerve dysfunction and stimulates angiogenesis in streptozotocin-diabetic rats. Diabetologia. 1992;35(1):12-8. Epub 1992/01/01.

[201] Kihara M, Mitsui MK, Mitsui Y, Okuda K, Nakasaka Y, Takahashi M, et al. Altered vasoreactivity to angiotensin II in experimental diabetic neuropathy: role of nitric oxide. Muscle Nerve. 1999;22(7):920-5. Epub 1999/07/09.

[202] Podar T, Tuomilehto J. The role of angiotensin converting enzyme inhibitors and angiotensin II receptor antagonists in the management of diabetic complications. Drugs. 2002;62(14):2007-12. Epub 2002/09/25.

[203] Malik RA, Williamson S, Abbott C, Carrington AL, Iqbal J, Schady W, et al. Effect of angiotensin-converting-enzyme (ACE) inhibitor trandolapril on human diabetic neuropathy: randomised double-blind controlled trial. Lancet. 1998;352(9145):1978-81. Epub 1999/01/01.

[204] Estacio RO, Jeffers BW, Gifford N, Schrier RW. Effect of blood pressure control on diabetic microvascular complications in patients with hypertension and type 2 diabetes. Diabetes care. 2000;23 Suppl 2:B54-64. Epub 2000/06/22.

[205] Tahrani AA, Askwith T, Stevens MJ. Emerging drugs for diabetic neuropathy. Expert opinion on emerging drugs. 2010;15(4):661-83. Epub 2010/08/28.

[206] Rivard A, Silver M, Chen D, Kearney M, Magner M, Annex B, et al. Rescue of diabetes-related impairment of angiogenesis by intramuscular gene therapy with adeno-VEGF. Am J Pathol. 1999;154(2):355-63. Epub 1999/02/23.

[207] Tsurumi Y, Takeshita S, Chen D, Kearney M, Rossow ST, Passeri J, et al. Direct intramuscular gene transfer of naked DNA encoding vascular endothelial growth factor

augments collateral development and tissue perfusion. Circulation. 1996;94(12): 3281-90. Epub 1996/12/15.

[208] Simovic D, Isner JM, Ropper AH, Pieczek A, Weinberg DH. Improvement in chronic ischemic neuropathy after intramuscular phVEGF165 gene transfer in patients with critical limb ischemia. Arch Neurol. 2001;58(5):761-8. Epub 2001/05/18.

[209] Baumgartner I, Pieczek A, Manor O, Blair R, Kearney M, Walsh K, et al. Constitutive expression of phVEGF165 after intramuscular gene transfer promotes collateral vessel development in patients with critical limb ischemia. Circulation. 1998;97(12): 1114-23. Epub 1998/04/16.

[210] Quattrini C, Jeziorska M, Boulton AJ, Malik RA. Reduced vascular endothelial growth factor expression and intra-epidermal nerve fiber loss in human diabetic neuropathy. Diabetes Care. 2008;31(1):140-5. Epub 2007/10/16.

[211] Lu M, Kuroki M, Amano S, Tolentino M, Keough K, Kim I, et al. Advanced glycation end products increase retinal vascular endothelial growth factor expression. J Clin Invest. 1998;101(6):1219-24. Epub 1998/04/29.

[212] Samii A, Unger J, Lange W. Vascular endothelial growth factor expression in peripheral nerves and dorsal root ganglia in diabetic neuropathy in rats. Neurosci Lett. 1999;262(3):159-62. Epub 1999/04/28.

[213] Chattopadhyay M, Krisky D, Wolfe D, Glorioso JC, Mata M, Fink DJ. HSV-mediated gene transfer of vascular endothelial growth factor to dorsal root ganglia prevents diabetic neuropathy. Gene Ther. 2005;12(18):1377-84. Epub 2005/04/22.

[214] Schratzberger P, Walter DH, Rittig K, Bahlmann FH, Pola R, Curry C, et al. Reversal of experimental diabetic neuropathy by VEGF gene transfer. J Clin Invest. 2001;107(9):1083-92. Epub 2001/05/09.

[215] Ropper AH, Gorson KC, Gooch CL, Weinberg DH, Pieczek A, Ware JH, et al. Vascular endothelial growth factor gene transfer for diabetic polyneuropathy: a randomized, double-blinded trial. Ann Neurol. 2009;65(4):386-93. Epub 2009/04/29.

[216] Veves A, King GL. Can VEGF reverse diabetic neuropathy in human subjects? J Clin Invest. 2001;107(10):1215-8. Epub 2001/05/26.

[217] http://www.natap.org/2009/newsUpdates/061009_02.htm. Analysis of Subjects with Moderately Severe Diabetic Neuropathy Shows Statistically Significant Improvement in Multiple Quantitative Neurological Endpoints2009.

[218] Eisenstein M. Sangamo's lead zinc-finger therapy flops in diabetic neuropathy. Nature Biotechnology [Internet]. 2012. Available from: http://www.nature.com.proxygw.wrlc.org/nbt/journal/v30/n2/full/nbt0212-121a.html.

[219] Horrobin DF. Essential fatty acids in the management of impaired nerve function in diabetes. Diabetes. 1997;46 Suppl 2:S90-3. Epub 1997/09/01.

[220] Mercuri O, Peluffo RO, Brenner RR. Depression of microsomal desaturation of linoleic to gamma-linolenic acid in the alloxan-diabetic rat. Biochim Biophys Acta. 1966;116(2):409-11. Epub 1966/04/04.

[221] Horrobin DF. The regulation of prostaglandin biosynthesis by the manipulation of essential fatty acid metabolism. Rev Pure Appl Pharmacol Sci. 1983;4(4):339-83. Epub 1983/10/01.

[222] Jones DB, Carter RD, Haitas B, Mann JI. Low phospholipid arachidonic acid values in diabetic platelets. Br Med J (Clin Res Ed). 1983;286(6360):173-5. Epub 1983/01/15.

[223] Arisaka M, Arisaka O, Fukuda Y, Yamashiro Y. Prostaglandin metabolism in children with diabetes mellitus. I. Plasma prostaglandin E2, F2 alpha, TXB2, and serum fatty acid levels. J Pediatr Gastroenterol Nutr. 1986;5(6):878-82. Epub 1986/11/01.

[224] Horrobin DF. The roles of essential fatty acids in the development of diabetic neuropathy and other complications of diabetes mellitus. Prostaglandins Leukot Essent Fatty Acids. 1988;31(3):181-97. Epub 1988/01/01.

[225] NINDS. Bethesda: National Institute of Neurological Disorders and Stroke; 2012.

[226] Head RJ, McLennan PL, Raederstorff D, Muggli R, Burnard SL, McMurchie EJ. Prevention of nerve conduction deficit in diabetic rats by polyunsaturated fatty acids. Am J Clin Nutr. 2000;71(1 Suppl):386S-92S. Epub 2000/01/05.

[227] Tomlinson DR, Robinson JP, Compton AM, Keen P. Essential fatty acid treatment--effects on nerve conduction, polyol pathway and axonal transport in streptozotocin diabetic rats. Diabetologia. 1989;32(9):655-9. Epub 1989/09/01.

[228] Julu PO. Essential fatty acids prevent slowed nerve conduction in streptozotocin diabetic rats. J Diabet Complications. 1988;2(4):185-8. Epub 1988/10/01.

[229] Cameron NE, Cotter MA. Interaction between oxidative stress and gamma-linolenic acid in impaired neurovascular function of diabetic rats. Am J Physiol. 1996;271(3 Pt 1):E471-6. Epub 1996/09/01.

[230] Jamal GA, Carmichael H. The effect of gamma-linolenic acid on human diabetic peripheral neuropathy: a double-blind placebo-controlled trial. Diabet Med. 1990;7(4): 319-23. Epub 1990/05/01.

[231] Keen H, Payan J, Allawi J, Walker J, Jamal GA, Weir AI, et al. Treatment of diabetic neuropathy with gamma-linolenic acid. The gamma-Linolenic Acid Multicenter Trial Group. Diabetes Care. 1993;16(1):8-15. Epub 1993/01/01.

[232] Takwale A, Tan E, Agarwal S, Barclay G, Ahmed I, Hotchkiss K, et al. Efficacy and tolerability of borage oil in adults and children with atopic eczema: randomised, double blind, placebo controlled, parallel group trial. Bmj. 2003;327(7428):1385. Epub 2003/12/13.

[233] Hoare C, Li Wan Po A, Williams H. Systematic review of treatments for atopic eczema. Health Technol Assess. 2000;4(37):1-191. Epub 2001/01/03.

[234] Dyer O. GMC reprimands doctor for research fraud. Bmj. 2003;326(7392):730.

[235] Barrett S. Primrose Oil and Eczema: How Research Was Promoted and Supressed2004. Available from: http://www.quackwatch.org/01QuackeryRelatedTopics/DSH/epo.html.

[236] Smith R. The drugs don't work. Br Med J (Clin Res Ed). 2003;327.

[237] Vincent AM, Russell JW, Low P, Feldman EL. Oxidative stress in the pathogenesis of diabetic neuropathy. Endocr Rev. 2004;25(4):612-28. Epub 2004/08/06.

[238] Obrosova IG. How does glucose generate oxidative stress in peripheral nerve? Int Rev Neurobiol. 2002;50:3-35. Epub 2002/08/30.

[239] Kasznicki J, Kosmalski M, Sliwinska A, Mrowicka M, Stanczyk M, Majsterek I, et al. Evaluation of oxidative stress markers in pathogenesis of diabetic neuropathy. Mol Biol Rep. 2012;39(9):8669-78. Epub 2012/06/22.

[240] Low PA, Nickander KK, Tritschler HJ. The roles of oxidative stress and antioxidant treatment in experimental diabetic neuropathy. Diabetes. 1997;46 Suppl 2:S38-42. Epub 1997/09/01.

[241] Schmeichel AM, Schmelzer JD, Low PA. Oxidative injury and apoptosis of dorsal root ganglion neurons in chronic experimental diabetic neuropathy. Diabetes. 2003;52(1):165-71. Epub 2002/12/28.

[242] Obrosova IG, Drel VR, Pacher P, Ilnytska O, Wang ZQ, Stevens MJ, et al. Oxidative-nitrosative stress and poly(ADP-ribose) polymerase (PARP) activation in experimental diabetic neuropathy: the relation is revisited. Diabetes. 2005;54(12):3435-41. Epub 2005/11/25.

[243] Sheetz MJ, King GL. Molecular understanding of hyperglycemia's adverse effects for diabetic complications. Jama. 2002;288(20):2579-88. Epub 2002/11/28.

[244] Collier A, Jackson M, Dawkes RM, Bell D, Clarke BF. Reduced free radical activity detected by decreased diene conjugates in insulin-dependent diabetic patients. Diabet Med. 1988;5(8):747-9. Epub 1988/11/01.

[245] Oberley LW. Free radicals and diabetes. Free Radic Biol Med. 1988;5(2):113-24. Epub 1988/01/01.

[246] Nickander KK, Schmelzer JD, Rohwer DA, Low PA. Effect of alpha-tocopherol deficiency on indices of oxidative stress in normal and diabetic peripheral nerve. J Neurol Sci. 1994;126(1):6-14. Epub 1994/10/01.

[247] Kumar A, Negi G, Sharma SS. Suppression of NF-kappaB and NF-kappaB regulated oxidative stress and neuroinflammation by BAY 11-7082 (IkappaB phosphorylation

inhibitor) in experimental diabetic neuropathy. Biochimie. 2012;94(5):1158-65. Epub 2012/02/22.

[248] Nagamatsu M, Nickander KK, Schmelzer JD, Raya A, Wittrock DA, Tritschler H, et al. Lipoic acid improves nerve blood flow, reduces oxidative stress, and improves distal nerve conduction in experimental diabetic neuropathy. Diabetes Care. 1995;18(8):1160-7. Epub 1995/08/01.

[249] Terada T, Hara K, Haranishi Y, Sata T. Antinociceptive effect of intrathecal administration of taurine in rat models of neuropathic pain. Can J Anaesth. 2011;58(7):630-7. Epub 2011/04/23.

[250] Firuzi O, Miri R, Tavakkoli M, Saso L. Antioxidant therapy: current status and future prospects. Curr Med Chem. 2011;18(25):3871-88. Epub 2011/08/10.

[251] Gemignani F. Symptomatic and pathogenetic treatment of diabetic neuropathy. Neural Regen Res. 2010;5(10):781-8.

[252] Ziegler D, Nowak H, Kempler P, Vargha P, Low PA. Treatment of symptomatic diabetic polyneuropathy with the antioxidant alpha-lipoic acid: a meta-analysis. Diabet Med. 2004;21(2):114-21. Epub 2004/02/27.

[253] Ziegler D, Low PA, Litchy WJ, Boulton AJ, Vinik AI, Freeman R, et al. Efficacy and safety of antioxidant treatment with alpha-lipoic acid over 4 years in diabetic polyneuropathy: the NATHAN 1 trial. Diabetes Care. 2011;34(9):2054-60. Epub 2011/07/22.

[254] Mijnhout GS, Alkhalaf A, Kleefstra N, Bilo HJ. Alpha lipoic acid: a new treatment for neuropathic pain in patients with diabetes? Neth J Med. 2010;68(4):158-62. Epub 2010/04/28.

[255] NINDS. In: Stroke DoHaHSNIoHNIoNDa, editor. Bethesda2012.

[256] Ziegler D, Luft D. Clinical trials for drugs against diabetic neuropathy: can we combine scientific needs with clinical practicalities? Int Rev Neurobiol. 2002;50:431-63. Epub 2002/08/30.

[257] Takano H, Nagai T, Asakawa M, Toyozaki T, Oka T, Komuro I, et al. Peroxisome proliferator-activated receptor activators inhibit lipopolysaccharide-induced tumor necrosis factor-alpha expression in neonatal rat cardiac myocytes. Circ Res. 2000;87(7):596-602. Epub 2000/09/29.

[258] Viberti GC. Rosiglitazone: potential beneficial impact on cardiovascular disease. Int J Clin Pract. 2003;57(2):128-34. Epub 2003/03/29.

[259] Nissen SE. The rise and fall of rosiglitazone. Eur Heart J. 2010;31(7):773-6. Epub 2010/02/16.

[260] Garcia M, Llames S, Garcia E, Meana A, Cuadrado N, Recasens M, et al. In vivo assessment of acute UVB responses in normal and Xeroderma Pigmentosum (XP-C) skin-humanized mouse models. Am J Pathol. 2010;177(2):865-72. Epub 2010/06/19.

[261] Olson H, Betton G, Robinson D, Thomas K, Monro A, Kolaja G, et al. Concordance of the toxicity of pharmaceuticals in humans and in animals. Regul Toxicol Pharmacol. 2000;32(1):56-67. Epub 2000/10/13.

[262] Topol EJ. Failing the public health--rofecoxib, Merck, and the FDA. N Engl J Med. 2004;351(17):1707-9. Epub 2004/10/08.

[263] Masubuchi Y. Metabolic and non-metabolic factors determining troglitazone hepatotoxicity: a review. Drug Metab Pharmacokinet. 2006;21(5):347-56. Epub 2006/10/31.

[264] Scientific Discussion. In: Agency EM, editor. London2005.

[265] Crivellente F. THE SOONER THE BETTER: utilising biomarkers to eliminate drug candidates with cardiotoxicity in preclinical development. Drug Discovery World. 2011 06/23:31-6.

[266] Ballard PA, Tetrud JW, Langston JW. Permanent human parkinsonism due to 1-methyl-4-phenyl-1,2,3,6-tetrahydropyridine (MPTP): seven cases. Neurology. 1985;35(7):949-56. Epub 1985/07/01.

[267] Langston JW. The Impact of MPTP on Parkinson's Disease Research: Past, Present, and Future. In: SA F, WJ W, editors. Parkinson's Disease: Diagnosis and Clinical Management. New York: Demos Medical Publishing; 2002.

[268] DM B. The Analgesic, Antipyretic and Anti-inflammatory Drugs. In: HR A, editor. Veterinary Pharmacology and Therapeutics. 8th ed. Iowa: Iowa University Press; 2001. p. 433-54.

[269] Shanks N, Greek R, Greek J. Are animal models predictive for humans? Philosophy, ethics, and humanities in medicine : PEHM. 2009;4:2. Epub 2009/01/17.

[270] Fox A, Eastwood C, Gentry C, Manning D, Urban L. Critical evaluation of the streptozotocin model of painful diabetic neuropathy in the rat. Pain. 1999;81(3):307-16. Epub 1999/08/04.

[271] Urban MJ, Li C, Yu C, Lu Y, Krise JM, McIntosh MP, et al. Inhibiting heat-shock protein 90 reverses sensory hypoalgesia in diabetic mice. ASN neuro. 2010;2(4). Epub 2010/08/17.

[272] Sullivan KA, Lentz SI, Roberts JL, Jr., Feldman EL. Criteria for creating and assessing mouse models of diabetic neuropathy. Curr Drug Targets. 2008;9(1):3-13. Epub 2008/01/29.

[273] Kamei J, Kawashima N, Narita M, Suzuki T, Misawa M, Kasuya Y. Reduction in ATP-sensitive potassium channel-mediated antinociception in diabetic mice. Psychopharmacology (Berl). 1994;113(3-4):318-21. Epub 1994/01/01.

[274] Levine AS, Morley JE, Wilcox G, Brown DM, Handwerger BS. Tail pinch behavior and analgesia in diabetic mice. Physiol Behav. 1982;28(1):39-43. Epub 1982/01/01.

[275] Pertovaara A, Wei H, Kalmari J, Ruotsalainen M. Pain behavior and response properties of spinal dorsal horn neurons following experimental diabetic neuropathy in the rat: modulation by nitecapone, a COMT inhibitor with antioxidant properties. Exp Neurol. 2001;167(2):425-34. Epub 2001/02/13.

[276] Courteix C, Bourget P, Caussade F, Bardin M, Coudore F, Fialip J, et al. Is the reduced efficacy of morphine in diabetic rats caused by alterations of opiate receptors or of morphine pharmacokinetics? J Pharmacol Exp Ther. 1998;285(1):63-70. Epub 1998/05/16.

[277] Lee JH, McCarty R. Pain threshold in diabetic rats: effects of good versus poor diabetic control. Pain. 1992;50(2):231-6. Epub 1992/08/01.

[278] Braiman-Wiksman L, Solomonik I, Spira R, Tennenbaum T. Novel insights into wound healing sequence of events. Toxicol Pathol. 2007;35(6):767-79. Epub 2007/10/19.

[279] Thomas PK. Diabetic neuropathy. Human and experimental. Drugs. 1986;32 Suppl 2:36-42. Epub 1986/01/01.

[280] Yagihashi S. Pathogenetic mechanisms of diabetic neuropathy: lessons from animal models. J Peripher Nerv Syst. 1997;2(2):113-32. Epub 1997/01/01.

[281] Yagihashi S, Kamijo M, Watanabe K. Reduced myelinated fiber size correlates with loss of axonal neurofilaments in peripheral nerve of chronically streptozotocin diabetic rats. Am J Pathol. 1990;136(6):1365-73. Epub 1990/06/01.

[282] Sima AA. The development and structural characterization of the neuropathies in the spontaneously diabetic BB Wistar rat. Metabolism. 1983;32(7 Suppl 1):106-11. Epub 1983/07/01.

[283] Sima AA, Hinton D. Hirano-bodies in the distal symmetric polyneuropathy of the spontaneously diabetic BB-Wistar rat. Acta Neurol Scand. 1983;68(2):107-12. Epub 1983/08/01.

[284] Uehara K, Sugimoto K, Wada R, Yoshikawa T, Marukawa K, Yasuda Y, et al. Effects of cilostazol on the peripheral nerve function and structure in STZ-induced diabetic rats. J Diabetes Complications. 1997;11(3):194-202. Epub 1997/05/01.

[285] Giannini C, Dyck PJ. Basement membrane reduplication and pericyte degeneration precede development of diabetic polyneuropathy and are associated with its severity. Ann Neurol. 1995;37(4):498-504. Epub 1995/04/01.

[286] Sima AA, Nathaniel V, Prashar A, Bril V, Greene DA. Endoneurial microvessels in human diabetic neuropathy. Endothelial cell dysjunction and lack of treatment effect by aldose reductase inhibitor. Diabetes. 1991;40(9):1090-9. Epub 1991/09/01.

[287] Sigaudo-Roussel D, Fromy B, Saumer JL. Diabetic Neuropathy in Animal Models. Drug Discovery Today: Disease Models. 2007;4:39-44.

[288] Adachi T, Yasuda K, Okamoto Y, Shihara N, Oku A, Ueta K, et al. T-1095, a renal Na +-glucose transporter inhibitor, improves hyperglycemia in streptozotocin-induced diabetic rats. Metabolism. 2000;49(8):990-5. Epub 2000/08/23.

[289] Ravi K, Ramachandran B, Subramanian S. Protective effect of Eugenia jambolana seed kernel on tissue antioxidants in streptozotocin-induced diabetic rats. Biol Pharm Bull. 2004;27(8):1212-7. Epub 2004/08/12.

[290] Assurance NCfQ. Diabetes Recognition Program (DRP). Washington, D.C.: National Committee for Quality Assurance; 2010 [cited 2012 10-20-2012]; Available from: http://www.ncqa.org/tabid/1023/Default.aspx.

[291] Gonzalez RG, Barnett P, Aguayo J, Cheng HM, Chylack LT, Jr. Direct measurement of polyol pathway activity in the ocular lens. Diabetes. 1984;33(2):196-9. Epub 1984/02/01.

[292] Urban MJ, Pan P, Farmer KL, Zhao H, Blagg BS, Dobrowsky RT. Modulating molecular chaperones improves sensory fiber recovery and mitochondrial function in diabetic peripheral neuropathy. Exp Neurol. 2012. Epub 2012/04/03.

[293] Usuki S, Ito Y, Morikawa K, Kise M, Ariga T, Rivner M, et al. Effect of pre-germinated brown rice intake on diabetic neuropathy in streptozotocin-induced diabetic rats. Nutr Metab (Lond). 2007;4:25. Epub 2007/11/27.

[294] Matsumoto T, Ono Y, Kurono M, Kuromiya A, Nakamura K, Bril V. Improvement of motor nerve conduction velocity in diabetic rats requires normalization of the polyol pathway metabolites flux. J Pharmacol Sci. 2009;109(2):203-10. Epub 2009/02/13.

[295] Malone JI, Lowitt S, Korthals JK, Salem A, Miranda C. The effect of hyperglycemia on nerve conduction and structure is age dependent. Diabetes. 1996;45(2):209-15. Epub 1996/02/01.

[296] Sherwood L. Principals of Neural and Hormonal Communication. In: Sherwood L, editor. Human Physiology: From Cells to Systems. 7th ed. Belmont: Brooks/Cole; 2008. p. 95.

[297] Cabrera O, Berman DM, Kenyon NS, Ricordi C, Berggren PO, Caicedo A. The unique cytoarchitecture of human pancreatic islets has implications for islet cell function. Proc Natl Acad Sci U S A. 2006;103(7):2334-9. Epub 2006/02/08.

[298] Molnar A, Borbely A, Czuriga D, Ivetta SM, Szilagyi S, Hertelendi Z, et al. Protein kinase C contributes to the maintenance of contractile force in human ventricular cardiomyocytes. J Biol Chem. 2009;284(2):1031-9. Epub 2008/10/16.

[299] Pelleymounter MA, Cullen MJ, Baker MB, Hecht R, Winters D, Boone T, et al. Effects of the obese gene product on body weight regulation in ob/ob mice. Science. 1995;269(5223):540-3. Epub 1995/07/28.

[300] Considine RV, Sinha MK, Heiman ML, Kriauciunas A, Stephens TW, Nyce MR, et al. Serum immunoreactive-leptin concentrations in normal-weight and obese humans. N Engl J Med. 1996;334(5):292-5. Epub 1996/02/01.

[301] Ras VR, Nava PB. Age-related changes of neurites in Meissner corpuscles of diabetic mice. Exp Neurol. 1986;91(3):488-501. Epub 1986/03/01.

Chapter 3

New Insights on Neuropathic Pain Mechanisms as a Source for Novel Therapeutical Strategies

Sabatino Maione, Enza Palazzo, Francesca Guida,
Livio Luongo, Dario Siniscalco, Ida Marabese,
Francesco Rossi and Vito de Novellis

Additional information is available at the end of the chapter

http://dx.doi.org/10.5772/55276

1. Introduction

Injuries affecting either the peripheral or the central nervous system (PNS, CNS) leads to neuropathic pain characterized by spontaneous pain and distortion or exaggeration of pain sensation. Peripheral nerve pathologies are considered generally easier to treat compared to those affecting the CNS, however peripheral neuropathies still remain a challenge to therapeutic treatment.

Animal models such as denervation/neuroma formation [1], chronic constriction injury (CCI) by loose ligatures around the sciatic nerve [2], partial tight ligation of the sciatic nerve trunk (partial sciatic nerve ligation, PNL) [3]; tight ligature of L5 and L6 spinal nerves (spinal nerve ligation, SNL) [4]; section of one or two components of the sciatic nerve (spared nerve injury, SNI) [5]; streptozocin induced diabetic neuropathy [6] and peripheral neuropathy induced by vincristine or by anti-retroviral nucleoside analogue AIDS therapy drugs [7, 8] have been designed to mimic different neuropathic syndromes and reproduce in laboratory neuropathic pain main symptoms. Indeed all the mentioned neuropathic pain models show increased responses to thermal or mechanical nociceptive stimulation (hyperalgesia), hypersensitivity to innocuous tactile or cold stimuli (allodynia) which lead to withdrawal behaviour.

2. Peripheral pathophysiology change mechanisms

A large body of studies has been accumulated during the last two decades to characterize and clarify mechanisms at the base of neuropathic pain development and maintenance. Peripheral nerve injury causes axon and myelin sheath degradation associated with macrophage, neutrophil and T cell infiltrations [9, 10].

The release of proinflammatory cytokines (interleukins, tumor necrosis factor-α) and mediators (bradykinins and prostaglandins) and growth factors (nerve growth factor) leads to peripheral sensitization and hypersensitivity to innocuous and noxious stimuli [11, 12]. Bradykinins and prostaglandins potentiates, among other things, the activity of transient receptor potential vanilloid type 1 (TRPV1) channel, highly expressed on Aδ and C fibers, whose activity and expression is potentiated in neuropathic pain models [13-16]. Neuropathic pain causes also over-expression of voltage gated sodium channels and increases sodium currents leading to spontaneous discharges of Aδ and C fibers [17-19]. Peripheral sensitization is also associated with increased voltage gated Ca^{2+} channels [20, 21]. Increased intracellular Ca^{2+} elevates substance P (SP) and glutamate release thus exacerbating pain transmission.

3. Spinal pathophysiology change mechanisms

Beside the peripheral mechanisms which are responsible of the immediate damage-induced changes in pain transmission, several spinal cellular and molecular changes are involved in the development of the neuropathic pain symptoms, such as thermal and mechanical hyperalgesia and tactile allodynia. Although first being thought as a disease of purely neuronal nature, several pre-clinical studies indicate that the mechanisms at the basis of the development and maintenance of neuropathic pain involve substantial contributions from the non-neuronal cells of both the PNS and CNS [22]. After peripheral nerve injury, microglia in the normal conditions (usually defined "resting" microglia) in the spinal dorsal horn proliferate and change their phenotype to an "activated" state through a series of cellular and molecular changes.

Microglia shift their phenotype to the hypertrophic "activated" form following altered expression of several molecules including cell surface receptors, intracellular signalling molecules and diffusible factors. The activation process consists of distinct cellular functions aimed at repairing damaged neural cells and eliminating debris from the damaged area [23]. Damaged cells release chemo-attractant molecules that both increase the motility (i.e. chemokinesis) and stimulate the migration (i.e. chemotaxis) of microglia, the combination of which recruits the microglia much closer to the damaged cells [24]. It has been shown that microglia activation in the spinal cord can be promoted by sciatic nerve ligation [25], spinal nerve ligation [26], sciatic nerve inflammation [27], traumatic nerve transection [28] and autoimmune diseases such as autoimmune encephalomyelitis and neuritis (EAE, EAN) [29, 30].

Once microglia become activated, they can exert both proinflammatory or anti-inflammatory/ neuroprotective functions depending on the combination of the stimulation of several receptors and the expression of specific genes [31]. Thus, the activation of microglia following a peripheral injury can be considered as an adaptation to tissue stress and malfunction [32] that contribute to the development and subsequent maintenance of chronic pain [33, 34].

http://dx.doi.org/10.5772/55276

Spinal microglia respond quickly to injury, up-regulating cell surface proteins and increasing synthesis and the release of inflammatory mediators, including cytokines and proteases that can sensitize neurons, thereby establishing positive feedback which helps to facilitate nociceptive signalling [35]. Accordingly, the inhibition of microglia targets can reduce hypersensitivity in neuropathic pain states.

The signals responsible for neuron-microglia and/or astrocyte communication are being extensively investigated since they may represent new targets for chronic pain management.

The first candidates are substances released by activated nociceptive primary afferent fibers, such as glutamate and SP, which are capable to activate microglia [36, 37]. Glutamate activates microglia by stimulating NMDA receptors [37], although other mechanisms involving metabotropic glutamate receptors (mGluRs) cannot be ruled out since it has been shown that mGluRs are expressed on microglial cells [38, 39]. SP acts mostly by activating microglia neurokinin-1 (NK1) receptors. Many mechanisms have been proposed for neuron-microglia crosstalk. Among these, the fractalkine (FKN, CX3CL1), a member of CX3C class of chemokines and its receptor CX3CR1 have been extensively investigated [39]. FKN is constitutively expressed by spinal cord and sensory neurons in the dorsal root ganglia (DRGs) [40-42], while CX3CR1 is exclusively expressed by microglia cells and, after peripheral nerve injury it is largely up-regulated in activated microglia [41]. FKN produces nociceptive behaviour by activating CX3CR1 on microglia and p38 mitogen-activated protein kinase (MAPK)-mediated pathways [42, 43]. A pathway for the cleavage of FKN from the membrane of neurons, has been elegantly demonstrated [42]. Briefly, neuronal FKN is cleaved by Cathepsin S (CatS), a proteolitic enzyme which is synthesized and released by activated microglia. Despite the CX3CL1/CX3CR1 pathway represents a pro-nociceptive non adaptive process, seems to perform also a neuro-protective action in neurodegenerative diseases [44].

Another chemokine implicated in neuron-glia communication is the chemokine (C-C motif) ligand 2 (CCL2, MCP-1), which is *de novo* expressed by sensory neurons as early as a day after peripheral injury [44]. Once released, CCL2 activates microglia via interaction with CCR2 receptors, and, accordingly, mice lacking CCR2 receptors display a reduction in nerve injury-induced tactile allodynia [45]. The action of the monocyte chemoattractant protein 1 (MCP-1) at the spinal level has also been demonstrated by the intrathecal administration of an MCP-1 neutralizing antibody, which proved able to inhibit neuropathic pain symptoms [44]. Another important candidate for neuronal-microglial cross-talk is ATP, that is produced by neurons as well as by glial cells. ATP exerts its effect on microglia by activating the purinergic ionotropic P2X4 and P2X7, as well as the metabotropic P2Y6 and P2Y12, receptors which are up and/or down-regulated in several conditions [46]. The stimulation of the P2X4 channel seems to be involved in the development of neuropathic pain by inducing the release of brain derived neurotrophic factor (BDNF) [47, 48]. In particular, this mechanism is believed to be responsible of the appearance of the tactile allodynia by inverting the ionic gradient of the GABAergic interneurons following the down-regulation of the KKC2 calcium transporter [47]. P2X4 receptor activation occurs earlier than that of P2X7 channel due to the greater affinity of ATP to bind to P2X4 receptor. Indeed, P2X7 is involved in the maintenance of microglial activation. The P2X7 receptor appears to be a functionally unique ionotropic receptor among the P2X receptor family since its activation is able to stimulate the release of the pro-inflammatory cytokine interleukin-1β (IL-1β) [49], as well as a variety of other pro-inflammatory cytokines. Recent studies have revealed that P2Y12R is also crucial in neuropathic pain induction and maintenance. It has been found that the expression of P2Y12R mRNA and protein are markedly enhanced in the spinal cord ipsilaterally to spinal nerve injury [50] or to sciatic nerve partial ligation [51]. The cellular location of this receptor in the spinal cord was highly restricted to microglia and recently has been proposed to be involved in the motility of microglial cell bodies and processes [52]. It is therefore possible that P2Y12R activity in microglia affects their ability to extend the branched processes toward neighbouring neurons of the pain matrix, which, in turn, may interfere with microglia-neuron communications. Recent data suggest that the metabotropic adenosine receptor A2A is also involved in the microglia process retraction occurring during microglia activation [53]. The up-regulation of Gs protein-coupled adenosine A2A receptor on activated microglia seems to occur concomitantly to down regulation of Gi-protein coupled P2Y12 receptor [53].

4. Supraspinal pathophysiology change mechanisms

Descending pain modulatory system undergoes morpho-functional changes following PNS or CNS injury contributing to neuropathic pain development and maintenance [54-56]. The pain modulatory centers include brainstem areas such as periacqueductal gray (PAG), locus cœreuleus (LC) and rostral ventromedial-medulla (RVM). PAG is recognised as a major source of pain inhibitory control: its activation produces hypoalgesia by inhibiting nociceptive sensory processing within the dorsal horn of the spinal cord [57, 58]. PAG-induced analgesia is produced through the activation of RVM consisting of the raphe magnus and its adjacent reticular nuclei. Different pain responding cell populations are found in RVM: ON, OFF and neutral cells. These cells show different reactions to nociceptive stimuli such as excitation, inhibition or irresponsiveness, respectively [59, 60]. Apart from their well-documented role in anti-nociception, PAG and RVM mediate also a descending facilitation [61, 62]. Indeed, a shift in the balance between RVM "pronociceptive" ON cells versus "antinociceptive" OFF cell activity has been found in neuropathic pain conditions. The ongoing firing of RVM ON cells was found significantly increased whereas the spontaneous activity of the OFF cells appeared decreased 7 days after neuropathic pain induction [60, 63]. A functional shift between ON and OFF cell activity such that ON cell activity predominates over that of the OFF may be responsible of the facilitatory influence of the RVM on spinal neurons leading to neuropathic hypersensitivity [64-66, 16, 67]. Moreover, a contribute of serotonergic neurons, considered a subset of neutral cells, in nociceptive modulation has been evidenced in abnormal pain states [68]. Thus, changes in RVM cell activity may be considered a sort of sensitization of RVM neurons during neuropathic pain [69, 70] as consequence of altered peripheral inputs associated with spinal processing [71]. Alternatively, RVM cell activity changes may reflect a different control exerted from the upstream PAG projections. Indeed, a complex morpho-functional reorganization has been observed within the PAG after neuropathic pain induction. A decrease in the potency of (R)-(+)-[2,3-dihydro-5-methyl-3-(4-morpholinylmethyl)pyrrolo[1,2,3-de]-1,4-benzoxazin-6-yl]-1-naphthalenylmethanonemesylate (WIN 55,212-2), a cannabinoid receptor agonist, locally microinjected into the ventrolateral (VL) PAG, has been recently evidenced in neuropathic rats. Seven days after the CCI of the sciatic nerve WIN 55,212-2 produced antinociception and inhibited the activity of the ON cells while increased those one of the OFF cells (as centrally acting analgesic drugs are expected to do) at doses twofold higher than in control rats [67]. Moreover, the expression of cannabinoid type 1 (CB1) receptor, the CB1 receptor associated Gαi3 and the cannabinoid receptor interacting 1a (CRIP 1a) proteins and the endocannabinoid synthesising enzyme NAPE-PLD proved to be decreased in CCI rats [67]. Thus a down regulation of the endocannabinoid system within the VL PAG, possibly due to endocannabinoid increase in neuropathic pain state [72], may lead to an enhancement in pain responses through an altered control of PAG-RVM circuitry on spinal nociceptive neurons. A hyperactivity of serotonergic neurons and an increase in endocannabinoids was also observed in CCI animals in dorsal raphe (DR), an area which lies just ventrally and shows similar morphological properties to the PAG [73]. DR phenotypic changes during neuropathic pain may have also relevance for the affective component of chronic pain. Another supraspinal circuitry being involved in to the emotional-affective aspects of pain is the basolateral amygdala (BLA)-medial prefrontal cortex (mPFC) pathway. Pyramidal neurons of mPFC respond to BLA electrical stimulation or hind-paw pressoceptive stimulation with an inhibitory [BLA→mPFC(-)] or excitatory [BLA→mPFC(+)] response [74]. These neurons show a phenotypic rearrangement in SNI-induced mono-neuropathy in the rat, suggesting that the mPFC may undergo profound reorganization in chronic pain conditions [75]. Neuropathic pain can shift the balance between excitatory and inhibitory responses in the BLA→mPFC pathway, resulting in a net increase in the excitatory influence that the BLA exerts over the prelimbic/infralimbic (PL/IL) neuron population of the mPFC [76-80]. These functional changes appeared concomitantly with an increase in glutamate levels, as well as an up-regulation of fatty acid amide hydrolase (FAAH) enzyme and TRPV1 channels in the PL/IL cortex of SNI rats [75]. Overexpression of several caspases such as caspase-3 and 1, upregulation of glutamate AMPA receptors in microglia, IL-1β and IL-1 receptor-1, TRPV1 and vesicular glutamate transporter 1 (VGluT1) in glutamatergic neurons were also observed 7 days after SNI in mice. Of these alterations, only those in astrocytes persisted in SNI TPRV1(-/-) mice. SNI triggers both TRPV1-dependent and independent glutamate- and caspase-mediated cross-talk among IL-PL cortex neurons and glia, which either participates or counteracts pain processing. Alterations in endovanilloid system associated with peripheral nerve injury may suggest that therapies able to normalize endovanilloid transmission or blocking caspase activation may prove useful in ameliorating symptoms and central sequelae associated with neuropathic pain [80, 75]. Within the VL PAG the expression of pronociceptive mediator targets such as the prostaglandin EP1 receptor, whose activation has pain facilitatory role, proved to be reduced 7 days after neuropathic pain induction by SNI. However, its blockade and stimulation was still able to inhibit/facilitate pain responses and the ON and OFF cell activity, as they did in control animals. The major expression of EP1 receptor was found on GABAergic neurons consistently with an EP1 receptor blockade-induced disinhibition of the antinociceptive descending pathway at VL PAG level and behavioural antinociception [16].

5. Cannabinoids and peripheral neuropathy

The discovery and characterization of cannabinoid receptors (CBRs) in the late eighties [81, 82] and the subsequent isolation of endogenous ligands, first of all the arachidonoylethanolamide (AEA) [83], established the existence of a proper endocannabinoid neuromodulatory system. Cannabinoids include the components of the cannabis plant (*Cannabis sativa L.*), the endogenous cannabinoids (endocannabinoids), and several synthetic cannabinoid ligands. The cannabinoid system is involved in several human physiological functions as testified by the fact that cannabis intake affects important aspects of behaviour such as short-term memory, panic reactions, motor coordination, food-intake and pain perception [84, 85]. More than 70 psychoactive compounds have been identified in cannabis, among which Δ^9-tetrahydrocannabinol (THC) accounting for most of the psychological and physical effects. Cannabinoids exert their effects through the activation of two G protein-coupled receptors identified as the cannabinoid CB1 and CB2. Their activation is associated with inhibition of adenylate cyclase and the stimulation of mitogen-activated protein kinase (MAPK). Moreover, CB1 receptor activation modulates calcium or potassium conductance properties linked to the reduction of neuronal excitability and neurotransmitter release [86]. CB1 receptor is wide expressed in the brain, including neuroanatomical regions subserving transmission and modulation of pain signals, such as the PAG, the RVM and the dorsal horn of the spinal cord [87, 88]. CB2 is found manly in the peripheral immune system. It is expressed on T and B cells, macrophages, natural killer and monocytes, however recent studies suggest its expression on neurons at dorsal root ganglia level and at central level within spinal cord, specifically on glia, microglia and neurons [89, 28]. Pharmacological evidence also support the existence of non–CB1/CB2 receptor-mediated cannabinoid effects [90] and different investigations have been identified possible targets in the orphan G protein–coupled receptor GPR55 [91], transient receptor potential vanilloid type-1 (TRPV1) channel [92] or peroxisome proliferator-activated receptors (PPARs) [93]. The endocannabinoids such as AEA, arachidonoylglycerol (2-AG) and *N*-arachidonoyl-dopamine (NADA) are lipid compounds produced *on demand* by the cleavage of membrane phospholipid precursors, released from cells immediately after their production and degraded by specific enzymatic system. AEA is synthesized from enzymatic cleavage of N-arachidonoyl phosphatidylethanolamine (NAPE) by a specific phospholipase D (NAPE-PLD). It shows higher affinity for CB (Ki [CB1 vs CB2] = 89 vs 371 nM) and can also activate ionotropic TRPV1 receptors as endovanilloids. Biological inactivation of anandamide occurs through a rapid uptake followed by intracellular hydrolysis mediated by FAAH.

2-AG, which is more abundant than anandamide in the brain binds to CB1 and CB2 with a lower affinity than anandamide, but behaves like a full agonist since it shows higher intrinsic activity [94]. 2-AG is synthesized by the enzyme diacylglycerol lipase (DGL-α) in a Ca^{2+}-dependent pathway [95]. Other alternative mechanisms of 2-AG synthesis have also been proposed [96]. Biological inactivation occurs through uptake followed by hydrolysis mediated by the enzyme monoacylglycerol lipase (MGL). Other enzymes have been indicated for 2-AG metabolism, including cyclooxygenases (COXs), lipooxygenases (LOXs) and FAAH [97, 98]. The first evidence of the analgesic properties of cannabis was observed in 1899 by Dixon [99]. Crucial studies on cannabinoid-induced antinociception by Bicher and Mechoulam (1968)

[100] and Kosersky [101] confirmed the ability of cannabinoids to inhibit acute and inflammatory and nerve injury–induced pain. Cannabinoids seem to be useful in alleviating neuropathic pain symptoms after prolonged treatments [102], unlike opioids, which show only limited effectiveness [103, 104]. The activation of the CB receptors by synthetic agonists, or pharmacological elevation of endocannabinoid levels, suppresses hyperalgesia and allodynia in animal models of neuropathic pain. Local administration of exogenous AEA or 2-AG significant decreases the hyperalgesia in formalin test or in the PNL [105, 106]. Systemic FAAH inhibitor (URB597, AA-5-HT, OL-135) administration or the inhibition of endocannabinoid uptake with AM404 produce antinociceptive effects in CCI [107] or PNL models [3] which are mainly CB1 receptor-mediated. It is also important to highlight that inhibitors of FAAH elevate levels of fatty-acid amides that do not bind to CB receptors (e.g. palmitoylethanolamine). Thus, the contribute of non-cannabinoid receptor mechanisms of action in the *in vivo* pharmacological effects of FAAH and MGL inhibitors must also be considered. Direct evidence for supraspinal sites of cannabinoid analgesic action was derived from the observation that administration of cannabinoids compounds straight into the brain induces antinociception. Martin et al. (1999) [108] demonstrated that WIN55,212-2 produced antinociception in the tail-flick test when injected into different brain regions including subnuclei of the amygdala, thalamus, PAG and RVM.

In addition, as previously briefly described, WIN55,212-2 microinjection into the PAG suppressed the sciatic nerve constriction-induced allodynia and modulated RVM cells activity [67]. Similar effects have been shown by intra-PAG injection of a FAAH inhibitor URB597 which elevates endocannabinoid levels and reduces the thermal nociception via activation of CB1 and TRPV1 receptor mechanisms [109]. Moreover, Giordano et al. (2011) [80] have shown that acute intra-pre-limbic/infra-limbic cortex microinjection of N-arachidonoyl-serotonin (AA-5-HT), a hybrid FAAH inhibitor and TPRV1 channel antagonist, transiently decreased the allodynia and modulates the changes occurring on cortex pyramidal neurons induced by SNI model.

In the complex scenario of neuropathic pain, which also involves non-neuronal pathways, such as microglial cell-induced synaptic plasticity, the endocannabinoid system may also represent target to exploite for modulating microglia-neuron communication. Several studies have focused on CB2 receptor activation in different neuropathic pain models [110, 28, 111, 112].

Such studies have highlighted the role of CB2 receptor in the modulation of immune response involved in the development of neuropathic pain. CB2 receptor activation exerts antiallodynic and antihyperalgesic effects by modulating microglia responses. In particular, CB2 receptor stimulation induced an analgesic effect in SNI mice associated with a reduction in the pro-inflammatory (IFN-γ and IL-1β) and an enhancement in anti-inflammatory (IL-10) mediators within the spinal cord [28]. Beside the analgesic effect, cannabis intake can impair cognitive and performance tasks, such as memory and learning [113]. Activation of central CB1 receptors lead to a combination of stimulatory and depressant effects [114]. Other effects including catalepsy, motor deficits and thermal imbalance have been observed after administration of centrally acting cannabinoids [115] These effects, mainly associated with activation of central CB1 receptors, deeply limit the clinical use of cannabinoids for the treatment of chronic pain states. The synthesis of CB2 receptor-selective agonists which lack of the majority of central side effects and produce antinociceptive effects represent an interesting pharmacological tool [116].

Cannabinoids can counteract pain in both physiological and pathological conditions. CB1Rs and CB2Rs are both overexpressed during inflammation and neuropathic pain. In this context, selective activation of peripheral CB1 or CB2 receptor by cannabinoid agents which do not penetrate the blood brain barriers or the enhancement of the endocannabinoid levels can be a promising therapeutic approach that avoid the side effects associated with central CB1 receptor activation. Finally the isolation of non psychotropic compounds of *Cannabis Sativa*, such as cannabidiol or cannabichromene, which show antinociceptive properties in physiological [117] and pathological [118] pain conditions, could represent an alternative tool in pain management.

6. Stem cell treatment for peripheral neuropathy

Management of peripheral neuropathy in affected patients could be tailored to individual requirements, for instance the presence of other co-morbidities could influence the therapy. Damaged peripheral nerves demonstrate some potential to regenerate, however, complete functional recovery is infrequent. Novel approaches are required in the clinical management of peripheral nerve injuries since the current surgical techniques result in deficient sensory recovery [119].

Nowadays, neuropathy research is focusing on newer cellular and molecular approaches, such as stem cell therapy. Preclinical studies indicate that stem cell therapy represents the great promise for the future of molecular and regenerative medicine, including tissue regeneration. In peripheral neuropathy, stem cells could act in several ways: i) improving the intrinsic regenerative capacity of injured nerves; ii) inhibiting pathogenic immune responses both in the periphery and inside the central nervous system; iii) releasing neuroprotective and anti-inflammatory molecules thus favouring tissue repair.

In the last years, it has been demonstrated that stem cells are neuroprotective in a variety of nervous system injury models [120]. Briefly, stem cells have been found in all multi-cellular organisms, they are able to divide and differentiate into diverse specialized cell types. In addition, stem cells self-renew themselves to produce more stem cells. Indeed, in principle, their extraordinary properties are the self-renewal (the ability to perform indefinite cell division cycles while maintaining the undifferentiated state) and the multipotency (the capacity to differentiate into specialized cell types). The availability of multiple stem cell types provides both the opportunity and a reasoned approach for treating several, otherwise untreatable, human diseases [121].

As neurodegenerative disease, also peripheral neuropathy could benefit by stem cell therapy. This cell- based treatment opportunity represents a non-surgical approaches to enhance nerve recovery and re-innervation processes [122, 123]. Indeed, stem cell implantation appears as a possible curative treatment having the stem cells the ability to incorporate into the site of a lesion, differentiate, and to improve locomotor recovery [124]. Stem cell beneficial effects are due to their properties, as self-renewal ability with the capacity to generate more identical stem cells; the capacity to give rise to more differentiated cells; the capacity to produce neuroprotective and anti-inflammatory molecules (paracrine regulatory functions) [121].

The ideal stem cell source for peripheral neuropathy repair should be easily accessible, involve non-invasive harvesting, be rapidly expandable in *in vitro* culture, be able to survive and integrate within the host nerve tissue [125]. Mesenchymal stem cells (MSCs) represent a promising therapeutic approach in nerve tissue engineering [126]. These cells are a population of progenitor cells of mesodermal origin found in the bone marrow of adults, giving rise to skeletal muscle cells, blood, adipose tissue, vascular and urogenital systems, and to connective tissues throughout the body [127]. This type of stem cells yields most prominent results in peripheral nerve re-generation. In addition, MSCs have great potential as therapeutic agents since they are easy to isolate and can be expanded from patients without serious ethical and technical problems [128]. MSC treatment into a polycaprolactone nerve guide was able to improve re-innervation and activity in mice undergone to nerve transection [129]. Interestingly, some transplanted stem cells assumed a Schwann-cell-like phenotype.

In a murine model of sciatic nerve crush injury, intravenous administration of adipose-derived MSC (ASC) significantly accelerated the functional recovery [126]. Mice showed significant improvement in fiber sprouting and the reduction of inflammatory infiltrates. The authors proposed that ASC-mediated positive effects were due to the production of *in situ* molecules, which, directly or indirectly through a cross-talk with local glia cells, could modulate the local environment with the down-regulation of inflammation and the promotion of axonal regeneration. Peripheral neuropathy is a dramatic symptom in Krabbe disease [130]. Hematopoietic stem cell (HSC) transplantation proved effective in slow the progression of this disease. HSCs were able to achieve improvement in peripheral nerve conduction abnormalities in Krabbe patients, suggesting remyelination of the nerves [131]. Diabetic neuropathy is the most common complication of diabetes, frequently leads to foot ulcers and may progress to limb amputations [132].

It has been proposed that autologous transplantation of bone marrow-derived mononuclear cells (BM-MNCs) could be a novel strategy for the treatment of painful diabetic neuropathy [133]. Indeed, transplantation of BM-MNCs is able to alleviate neuropathic pain in the early stage of streptozotocin-induced diabetic rats. The BM-MNC transplantation significantly ameliorated mechanical hyperalgesia and cold allodynia. Diabetic neuropathy is attracting most research strategies. Several clinical trials have been performed on the use of stem cells for the treatment of human peripheral diabetic neuropathy (www.clinicaltrials.gov). Induced pluripotent stem (iPS) cell technology has enormous potentials to advance medical therapy by personalizing regenerative medicine [134]. iPS cells offer great potentials as a future tool also for the treatment of peripheral neuropathy. Cell incorporation into conduit repair of peripheral nerves demonstrates experimental promise as a novel intervention. Tissue-engineered bioabsorbable nerve conduits coated with iPS cell-derived neurospheres were able to repair peripheral nerve gaps in mice [135].

Achieving peripheral nerve regeneration, axonal regeneration and re-myelination with stem cells is a challenging research goal. This process is very complex, with Wallerian degeneration being the most elementary reaction and Schwann cells playing an important role. An emerging solution to improve upon this intrinsic regenerative capacity is to supplement injured nerves with stem cells [136]. Stem cells effectiveness in the treatment of peripheral nerve injury may lie in their ability to differentiate into Schwann cells, secrete neurotrophic factors, and assist in myelin formation [137, 136]. This strategy of introduction autologous stem cells directly into the site of a nerve injury represents a promising therapy. Skin-derived precursor cells (SKPs) were successfully transplanted in the sciatic nerve of Lewis rats bridged by a freeze-thawed nerve graft.

The cells were able to improve nerve re-generation, probably their effect was due to the ability to secrete bioactive neurotrophins [138]. Another stem cell type, the multipotent hair follicle stem cells, could provide a potential accessible, autologous source of stem cells for regeneration therapy of damaged nerves [139]. More recently, in an interesting study, Amoh et al. transplanted hair follicle stem cells around the impinged sciatic nerve of the mice. The cells differentiated into glia fibrillary acidic protein-positive Schwann cells, promoting the recovery of pre-existing axons. Authors reported that the regenerated sciatic nerve was functionally recovered [140]. These hair follicle stem cells could differentiate into several cell types, i.e. neurons, glia, keratinocytes, smooth muscle cells and melanocytes. They are nestin-positive cells and once implanted into the gap region of the sciatic or tibial nerve, are able to enhance the rate of nerve regeneration and the restoration of nerve function [141]. Wharton's jelly fish-derived mesenchymal stem cells (WJMSCs) could be also a promising cell source for nerve tissue engineering. It has been demonstrated that these cells can be differentiated into Schwann-like cells and could be suitable Schwann-cell substitutes for nerve repair in clinical applications [142]. A recent strategy for peripheral nerve regeneration is based on the use of CD34(+) cells. Indeed, integration of CD34(+) cells in injured nerve significantly promotes nerve regeneration [143]. However, limited migration and short survival of CD34(+) cells could counteract this beneficial effect. One strategy could be the potentiation of CD34(+) cell recruitment triggered by stromal cell-derived factor-1α (SDF-1α) [143]. This strategy based on the over-expression of SDF-1α is providing interesting results in the peripheral neuropathy treatment. It has been proposed that the expression of SDF-1α in the injured nerve exerts a trophic effect by recruiting progenitor cells that promote nerve regeneration. Intravenous administration of human amniotic fluid-derived mesenchymal stem cells facilitated neural regeneration in a sciatic nerve crush injury model, when recruited by expression of SDF-1α in muscle and nerve after nerve crush injury [144]. As mesenchymal stem cells, amniotic fluid-derived mesenchymal stem cells have the ability to secrete neurotrophic factors that are able to promote neuron survival. Their transplantation was able to regenerate the sciatic nerve after crush injury by secretion of neurotrophic factors [145]. Interestingly, the stem cell mediated effects could be enhanced by co-administration of several anti-inflammatory and antiapoptotic factors, i.e. fermented soybean extracts or granulocyte-colony stimulating factor (G-CSF) [146, 147].

In some cases, stem cell therapy does not provide optimal results. The multipotent capacity of stem cells to differentiate into many cell types has led to successful therapy, but concerns remain about the possible negative or harmful effects of the transplanted cultured cells [148]. Mahdi-Rogers et al. treated six patients with chronic acquired demyelinating neuropathy with autologous peripheral blood stem cell transplantation (PBSCT) [149]. These patients were refractory to other treatments; however, the authors reported serious adverse events and lack of sustained response. There have been reports of inflammatory peripheral neuropathy or polyneuropathy associated with chronic graft-versus-host disease (GVHD) [150], even if pathogenesis has not been fully cleared. Doi et al. report a case of immune-mediated neuropathy after allogenic hematopoietic stem cell transplantation for Philadelphia-chromosome-positive acute lymphoblastic leukemia [151].On the other hand, a case of peripheral neuropathy induction was reported after autologous blood stem cell transplantation for multiple myeloma [152]. Overall, these data indicate that before being suitable for clinical applications, stem cell biology needs to be investigated further and in greater detail [153].

7. Conclusions

Neuropathic pain involves a complex network of mechanisms involving peripheral and central nervous system. The peripheral nerve injury produces abnormal peripheral afferent inputs at the spinal dorsal horn which leads to development of central sensitization and plastic changes in supraspinal areas. The precise contribute of the different brain sites in neuropathic pain development and maintenance is still far to be established. In particular the contribute of the descending pain modulatory system including the PAG and the RVM is dual varying from inhibitory to facilitatory. By this subject strategies able to shift the balance between facilitatory versus inhibitory influences of the descending pathway may be useful to counteract neuropathic pain symptoms. Cannabinoids have been proved to stimulate the PAG-RVM inhibitory pain control and inhibit neuropathic pain-related allodynia and hyperalgesia.

Neurons are not the only cell type involved in plastic changes at the base of pain hypersensitivity and activated microglia actively contribute to pain facilitation through a tight interaction with neuron activity and the release of pain mediators. Novel strategies based on switching off the microglia activation represents a possible therapeutic intervention to alleviate neuropathic pain.

Human mesenchymal stem cell transplantation has shown to reduce astrocytic and microglial cell activation, mechanical allodynia and cellular and molecular pain mechanisms. The therapeutic potentiality of stem cell to alleviate neuropathic pain appears encouraging, however, its clinical application in peripheral neuropathy requires and deserves further investigations.

Author details

Sabatino Maione, Enza Palazzo, Francesca Guida, Livio Luongo, Dario Siniscalco, Ida Marabese, Francesco Rossi and Vito de Novellis

Department of Experimental Medicine, Division of Pharmacology, Second University of Naples, Naples, Italy

References

[1] Wall, P. D, Devor, M, Inbal, R, Scadding, J. W, Schonfeld, D, Seltzer, Z, & Tomkiewicz, M. M. Autotomy following peripheral nerve lesions: experimental anaesthesia dolorosa. Pain (1979). , 7(2), 103-11.

[2] Bennett, G. J, & Xie, Y. K. A peripheral mononeuropathy in rat that produces disorders of pain sensation like those seen in man. Pain (1988). , 33(1), 87-107.

[3] Seltzer, Z, Dubner, R, & Shir, Y. A novel behavioral model of neuropathic pain disorders produced in rats by partial sciatic nerve injury. Pain (1990). , 43(2), 205-18.

[4] Kim, S. H, & Chung, J. M. (1992). An experimental model for peripheral neuropathy produced by segmental spinal nerve ligation in the rat. Pain , 50, 355-363.

[5] Decosterd, I, & Woolf, C. J. Spared nerve injury: an animal model of persistent peripheral neuropathic pain. Pain (2000). , 87(2), 149-58.

[6] Courteix, C, Bardin, M, Chantelauze, C, Lavarenne, J, & Eschalier, A. Study of thesensitivity of the diabetes-induced pain model in rats to a range of analgesics. Pain (1994). , 57(2), 153-60.

[7] Higuera, E. S, & Luo, Z. D. A rat pain model of vincristine-induced neuropathy. Methods Mol Med. (2004). , 99, 91-8.

[8] Joseph, E. K, Chen, X, Khasar, S. G, & Levine, J. D. Novel mechanism of enhanced nociception in a model of AIDS therapy-induced painful peripheral neuropathy in the rat. Pain (2004).

[9] Moalem, G, & Tracey, D. J. Immune and inflammatory mechanisms in neuropathic pain. Brain Res Rev (2006). , 51(2), 240-64.

[10] Scholz, J, & Woolf, C. J. The neuropathic pain triad: neurons, immune cells and glia. Nat Neurosci (2007). , 10, 1361-1368.

[11] Sommer, C, & Kress, M. Recent findings on how proinflammatory cytokines cause pain: peripheral mechanisms in inflammatory and neuropathic hyperalgesia. Neurosci Lett. (2004).

[12] Pezet, S, & Mcmahon, S. B. Neurotrophins: mediators and modulators of pain. Annu Rev Neurosci. (2006). , 29, 507-38.

[13] Hudson, L. J, Bevan, S, Wotherspoon, G, Gentry, C, Fox, A, & Winter, J. VR1 protein expression increases in undamaged DRG neurons after partial nerve injury. Eur J Neurosci (2001). , 13(11), 2105-14.

[14] Levine, J. D, & Alessandri-haber, N. TRP channels: targets for the relief of pain. Biochim Biophys Acta (2007). , 1772(8), 989-1003.

[15] Palazzo, E, Luongo, L, De Novellis, V, Berrino, L, Rossi, F, & Maione, S. Moving towards supraspinal TRPV1 receptors for chronic pain relief. Mol Pain (2010).

[16] Palazzo, E, Guida, F, Gatta, L, Luongo, L, Boccella, S, Bellini, G, Marabese, I, De Novellis, V, Rossi, F, & Maione, S. EP1 receptor within the ventrolateral periaqueductal grey controls thermonociception and rostral ventromedial medulla cell activity in healthy and neuropathic rat. Mol Pain (2011).

[17] Woolf, C. J, & Mannion, R. J. Neuropathic pain: Aetiology, symptoms, mechanisms, and management. Lancet (1999). , 353(9168), 1959-64.

[18] Hong, S, Morrow, T. J, Paulson, P. E, Isom, L. L, & Wiley, J. W. Early painful diabetic neuropathy is associated with differential changes in tetrodotoxin-sensitive and-resistant sodium channels in dorsal root ganglion neurons in the rat. J Biol Chem (2004). , 279(28), 29341-50.

[19] Hong, S, & Wiley, J. W. Early painful diabetic neuropathy is associated with differential changes in the expression and function of vanilloid receptor 1. J Biol Chem (2005). , 280(1), 618-27.

[20] Luo, Z. D, Chaplan, S. R, Higuera, E. S, Sorkin, L. S, Stauderman, K. A, Williams, M. E, & Yaksh, T. L. Upregulation of dorsal root ganglion (alpha)2(delta) calcium channel subunit and its correlation with allodynia in spinal nerve-injured rats. J Neurosci (2001). , 21(6), 1868-75.

[21] Matthews, E. A, & Dickenson, A. H. Effects of spinally delivered N- and P-type voltage-dependent calcium channel antagonists on dorsal horn neuronal responses in a rat model of neuropathy. Pain (2001).

[22] Scholz, J. Woolf CJ: The neuropathic pain triad: neurons, immune cells and glia. Nat Neurosci (2007).

[23] Garden, G. A, & Moller, T. Microglia biology in health and disease. J Neuroimmune Pharmacol (2006). , 1, 127-137.

[24] Trapp, B. D, Wujek, J. R, Criste, G. A, et al. Evidence for synaptic stripping by cortical microglia. Glia (2007). , 55, 360-368.

[25] Coyle, D. E. Partial peripheral nerve injury leads to activation of astroglia and microglia which parallels the development of allodynic behavior. Glia (1998). , 23(1), 75-83.

[26] Jin, S. X, Zhuang, Z. Y, Woolf, C. J, & Ji, R. R. p38 mitogen-activated protein kinase is activated after a spinal nerve ligation in spinal cord microglia and dorsal root ganglion neurons and contributes to the generation of neuropathic pain. J Neurosci (2003). , 23(10), 4017-22.

[27] Ledeboer, A, Sloane, E. M, Milligan, E. D, et al. Minocycline attenuates mechanical allodynia and proinflammatory cytokine expression in rat models of pain facilitation. Pain (2005).

[28] Luongo, L, Palazzo, E, Tambaro, S, et al. 1-(2',4'-dichlorophenyl)-6- methyl-N-cyclohexylamine-1,4-dihydroindeno[1,2-c]pyrazole-3- carboxamide, a novel CB2 agonist, alleviates neuropathic pain through functional microglial changes in mice. Neurobiol Dis (2010). , 37, 177-85.

[29] Olechowski, C. J, Truong, J. J, & Kerr, B. J. Neuropathic pain behaviours in a chronic-relapsing model of experimental autoimmune encephalomyelitis (EAE). Pain (2009).

[30] Luongo, L, Sajic, M, Grist, J, Clark, A. K, Maione, S, & Malcangio, M. Spinal changes associated with mechanical hypersensitivity in a model of Guillain-Barré syndrome. Neurosci Lett (2008). , 437(2), 98-102.

[31] Stella, N. Endocannabinoid signaling in microglial cells. Neuropharmacology (2009). Suppl , 1, 244-53.

[32] Medzhitov, R. Origin and physiological roles of inflammation. Nature (2008). , 454(7203), 428-35.

[33] Romero-sandoval, A. Nutile-McMenemy N, DeLeo JA. Spinal microglial and perivascular cell cannabinoid receptor type 2 activation reduces behavioral hypersensitivity without tolerance after peripheral nerve injury. Anesthesiology (2008). , 108(4), 722-734.

[34] Milligan, E. D, & Watkins, L. R. Pathological and protective roles of glia in chronic pain. Nat Rev Neurosci (2009). , 10(1), 23-36.

[35] Abbadie, C, Bhangoo, S, De Koninck, Y, Malcangio, M, Melik- Parsadaniantz, S, & White, F. A. Chemokines and pain mechanisms. Brain Res Rev (2009). , 60(1), 125-34.

[36] Lever, I. J, Bradbury, E. J, Cunningham, J. R, et al. Brain-derived neurotrophic factor is released in the dorsal horn by distinctive patterns of afferent fiber stimulation. J Neurosci (2001). , 21, 4469-4477.

[37] Svensson, C. I, Hua, X. Y, Protter, A. A, Powell, H. C, Yaksh, T. L, & Spinal, p. MAP kinase is necessary for NMDA-induced spinal PGE(2) release and thermal hyperalgesia. Neuroreport (2003a). , 14, 1153-1157.

[38] Taylor, D. L, Diemel, L. T, & Pocock, J. M. Activation of microglial group III metabotropic glutamate receptors protects neurons against microglial neurotoxicity. J Neurosci (2003). , 23(6), 2150-60.

[39] Biber, K, Laurie, D. J, Berthele, A, et al. Expression and signaling of group I metabotropic glutamate receptors in astrocytes and microglia. J Neurochem (1999). , 72(4), 1671-80.

[40] Bazan, J. F, Bacon, K. B, Hardiman, G, et al. A new class of membrane- bound chemokine with a CX3C motif. Nature (1997). , 385, 640-644.

[41] Lindia, J. A, Mcgowan, E, Jochnowitz, N, & Abbadie, C. Induction of CX3CL1 expression in astrocytes and CX3CR1 in microglia in the spinal cord of a rat model of neuropathic pain. J Pain (2005). , 6, 434-438.

[42] Clark, A. K, Yip, P. K, Grist, J, et al. Inhibition of spinal microglial cathepsin S for the reversal of neuropathic pain. Proc Natl Acad Sci USA (2007). , 104, 10655-10660.

[43] Zhuang, ZY, Kawasaki, Y, Tan, PH, & Wen, . . Role of the CX3CR1/p38 MAPK pathway in spinal microglia for the development of neuropathic pain following nerve injury-induced cleavage of fractalkine. Brain Behav Immun 2007; 21: 642- 651

[44] Thacker, M. A, Clark, A. K, Bishop, T, et al. CCL2 is a key mediator of microglia activation in neuropathic pain states. Eur J Pain (2009). , 13, 263-272.

[45] Abbadie, C, Lindia, J. A, Cumiskey, A. M, et al. Impaired neuropathic pain responses in mice lacking the chemokine receptor CCR2. Proc Natl Acad Sci USA (2003). , 100, 7947-7952.

[46] Inoue, K, Tsuda, M, & Tozaki-saitoh, H. Modification of neuropathic pain sensation through microglial ATP receptors. Purinergic Signal (2007). , 3, 311-316.

[47] Coull, J. A, Beggs, S, Boudreau, D, et al. BDNF from microglia causes the shift in neuronal anion gradient underlying neuropathic pain. Nature (2005). , 438, 1017-1021.

[48] Ulmann, L, Hatcher, J. P, Hughes, J. P, et al. Up-regulation of receptors in spinal microglia after peripheral nerve injury mediates BDNF release and neuropathic pain. J Neurosci (2008). , 2X4.

[49] Clark, A. K, Wodarski, R, Guida, F, Sasso, O, & Malcangio, M. Cathepsin S release from primary cultured microglia is regulated by the receptor. Glia (2010). , 2X7.

[50] Tozaki-saitoh, H, Tsuda, M, Miyata, H, Ueda, K, Kohsaka, S, & Inoue, K. P. Y12 receptors in spinal microglia are required for neuropathic pain after peripheral nerve injury. J Neurosci (2008). , 28(19), 4949-56.

[51] Kobayashi, K, Yamanaka, H, Fukuoka, T, Dai, Y, Obata, K, & Noguchi, K. P. Y12 receptor upregulation in activated microglia is a gateway of signaling and neuropathic pain. J Neurosci (2008). , 38.

[52] Haynes, S. E, Hollopeter, G, Yang, G, et al. The 2Y12 receptor regulates microglial activation by extracellular nucleotides. Nat Neurosci (2006).

[53] Orr, A. G, Orr, A. L, Li, X. J, Gross, R. E, Traynelis, S. F, & Adenosine, A. A) receptor mediates microglial process retraction. Nat Neurosci (2009). , 12(7), 872-8.

[54] Pertovaara, A. Plasticity in descending pain modulatory systems. Prog Brain Res (2000). , 129, 231-42.

[55] Porreca, F, Ossipov, M. H, & Gebhart, G. F. Chronic pain and medullary descending facilitation. Trends Neurosci. (2002). , 25(6), 319-25.

[56] Ossipov, M. H, & Porreca, F. Chapter 14 Descending excitatory systems. Handb Clin Neurol. (2006). , 81, 193-210.

[57] Reynolds, D. V. Surgery in the rat during electrical analgesia induced by focal brain stimulation. Science (1969). Apr 25;, 164(3878), 444-5.

[58] Jones, S. L, & Gebhart, G. F. Inhibition of spinal nociceptive transmission from the midbrain, pons and medulla in the rat: activation of descending inhibition by morphine, glutamate and electrical stimulation. Brain Res (1988).

[59] Fields, H. L, Bry, J, Hentall, I, & Zorman, G. The activity of neurons in the rostral medulla of the rat during withdrawal from noxious heat. J Neurosci. (1983).

[60] Fields, H. L, Basbaum, A. I, & Heinricher, M. M. (2006). Central nervous system mechanisms of pain modulation. In Mcmahon, SB and Kolzenburg M (Eds), Wall and Melzack's textbook of pain, 5th edn. Elsevier Location, China, , 125-142.

[61] Gebhart, G. F. Descending modulation of pain. Neurosci Biobehav Rev. (2004). Jan;, 27(8), 729-37.

[62] Vanegas, H, & Schaible, H. G. Descending control of persistent pain: inhibitory or facilitatory? Brain Res Brain Res Rev. (2004). , 46(3), 295-309.

[63] Gonçalves, L, Almeida, A, & Pertovaara, A. Pronociceptive changes in response properties of rostroventromedial medullary neurons in a rat model of peripheral neuropathy. Eur J Neurosci (2007). , 26(8), 2188-95.

[64] Kovelowski, C. J, Ossipov, M. H, Sun, H, Lai, J, Malan, T. P, & Porreca, F. Supraspinal cholecystokinin may drive tonic descending facilitation mechanisms to maintain neuropathic pain in the rat. Pain (2000). , 87(3), 265-73.

[65] Porreca, F, Burgess, S. E, Gardell, L. R, & Vanderah, T. W. Malan TP Jr, Ossipov MH, Lappi DA, Lai J. Inhibition of neuropathic pain by selective ablation of brainstem medullary cells expressing the mu-opioid receptor. J Neurosci. (2001). , 21(14), 5281-8.

[66] Carlson, J. D, Maire, J. J, Martenson, M. E, & Heinricher, M. M. Sensitization of pain-modulating neurons in the rostral ventromedial medulla after peripheral nerve injury. J Neurosci (2007). , 27(48), 13222-31.

[67] Palazzo, E, Luongo, L, Bellini, G, Guida, F, Marabese, I, Boccella, S, Rossi, F, Maione, S, & De Novellis, V. Changes in cannabinoid receptor subtype 1 activity and interaction with metabotropic glutamate subtype 5 receptors in the periaqueductal gray-ros-

tral ventromedial medulla pathway in a rodent neuropathic pain model. CNS Neurol Disord Drug Targets. (2012). , 2012(11), 148-61.

[68] Suzuki, R, Rygh, L. J, & Dickenson, A. H. Bad news from the brain: descending 5-HT pathways that control spinal pain processing. Trends Pharmacol. Sci. (2004). , 25, 613-617.

[69] Millecamps, M, Centeno, M. V, Berra, H. H, Rudick, C. N, Lavarello, S, & Tkatch, T. Apkarian AV. D-cycloserine reduces neuropathic pain behavior through limbic NMDA-mediated circuitry. Pain (2007).

[70] Tracey, I, & Mantyh, P. W. The cerebral signature for pain perception and its modulation. Neuron. (2007). , 55(3), 377-91.

[71] Campbell, J. N, & Meyer, R. A. Mechanisms of neuropathic pain. Neuron (2006). , 52(1), 77-92.

[72] Petrosino, S, Palazzo, E, De Novellis, V, Bisogno, T, Rossi, F, & Maione, S. Di Marzo V. Changes in spinal and supraspinal endocannabinoid levels in neuropathic rats. Neuropharmacology (2007). , 52(2), 415-22.

[73] Palazzo, E, De Novellis, V, Petrosino, S, Marabese, I, Vita, D, & Giordano, C. Di Marzo V, Mangoni GS, Rossi F, Maione S. Neuropathic pain and the endocannabinoid system in the dorsal raphe: pharmacological treatment and interactions with the serotonergic system. Eur J Neurosci. (2006). , 24(7), 2011-20.

[74] Floresco, S. B, & Tse, M. T. Dopaminergic regulation of inhibitory and excitatory transmission in the basolateral amygdala-prefrontal cortical pathway. J Neurosci. (2007). Feb 21;, 27(8), 2045-57.

[75] De Novellis, V, Vita, D, Gatta, L, Luongo, L, Bellini, G, De Chiaro, M, Marabese, I, Siniscalco, D, Boccella, S, & Piscitelli, F. Di Marzo V, Palazzo E, Rossi F, Maione S. The blockade of the transient receptor potential vanilloid type 1 and fatty acid amide hydrolase decreases symptoms and central sequelae in the medial prefrontal cortex of neuropathic rats. Mol Pain (2011). , 17, 7-7.

[76] Fu, Y, & Neugebauer, V. Differential mechanisms of CRF1 and CRF2 receptor functions in the amygdala in pain-related synaptic facilitation and behavior. J Neurosci. 20089;, 28(15), 3861-76.

[77] Neugebauer, V, Galhardo, V, Maione, S, & Mackey, S. C. Forebrain pain mechanisms. Brain Res Rev (2009). , 60(1), 226-42.

[78] Ji, G, & Neugebauer, V. Hemispheric lateralization of pain processing by amygdala neurons. J Neurophysiol (2009). , 102(4), 2253-64.

[79] Metz, A. E, Yau, H. J, Centeno, M. V, Apkarian, A. V, & Martina, M. Morphological and functional reorganization of rat medial prefrontal cortex in neuropathic pain. Proc Natl Acad Sci U S A (2009). , 106(7), 2423-8.

[80] Giordano, C, Cristino, L, Luongo, L, Siniscalco, D, Petrosino, S, Piscitelli, F, Marabese, I, Gatta, L, Rossi, F, Imperatore, R, Palazzo, E, & De Novellis, V. Di Marzo V, Maione S. Cereb Cortex (2011). in press

[81] Matsuda, L. A, Lolait, S. J, Brownstein, M. J, Young, A. C, & Bonner, T. I. Structure of a cannabinoid receptor and functional expression of the cloned cDNA. Nature (1990). , 346, 561-564.

[82] Herkenham, M, Lynn, A. B, Johnson, M. R, Melvin, L. S, De Costa, B. R, & Rice, K. C. Characterization and localization of cannabinoid receptors inrat brain: a quantitative in vitro autoradiographic study J Neurosci(1991). , 1, 563-583.

[83] Devane, W. A, Hanus, L, Breuer, A, et al. Isolation and structure of a brain constituent that binds to the cannabinoid receptor Science (1992). , 258, 1946-1949.

[84] Fride, E, Bregman, T, & Kirkham, T. C. Endocannabinoids and food intake: newborn suckling and appetite regulation in adulthood. Exp Biol Med (2005). Review., 230(4), 225-34.

[85] Guindon, J, & Hohmann, A. G. The endocannabinoid system and pain.CNS Neurol Disord Drug Targets. (2009). Review., 8(6), 403-21.

[86] Howlett, A. C. Cannabinoid receptor signaling. Handb. Exp. Pharmacol (2005). , 168, 53-79.

[87] Bushlin, I, Rozenfeld, R, & Devi, L. A. Cannabinoid-opioid interactions during neuropathic pain and analgesia. Curr Opin Pharmacol. (2010). , 10(1), 80-6.

[88] Miller, L. K, & Devi, L. A. The highs and lows of cannabinoid receptor expression in disease: mechanisms and their therapeutic implications. Pharmacol Rev. (2011). , 63(3), 461-70.

[89] Van Sickle, M. D, Duncan, M, Kingsley, P. J, Mouihate, A, Urbani, P, Mackie, K, Stella, N, Makriyannis, A, Piomelli, D, Davison, J. S, & Marnett, L. J. Di Marzo V, Pittman QJ, Patel KD, Sharkey KA. Identification and functional characterization of brainstem cannabinoid CB2 receptors Science (2005). , 310, 329-332.

[90] Staton PC, Hatcher JP, Walker DJ, Morrison AD, Shapland EM, Hughes JP, Chong E, Mander PK, Green PJ, Billinton A, Fulleylove M, Lancaster HC, Smith JC, Bailey LT, Wise A, Brown AJ

[91] Sharir, H. and Abood, M.E. Pharmacological characterization of GPR55, a putative cannabinoid receptor Pharmacol. Ther 2010;126(3):301–313

[92] Zygmunt, P. M, Petersson, J, Andersson, D. A, Chuang, H, & Sorgard, M. Di Marzo, V., Julius, D., and Hogestatt, E.D. Vanilloid receptors on sensory nerves mediate the vasodilator action of anandamide Nature (1999). , 400(6743), 452-457.

[93] Sullivan, O. S.E. Cannabinoids go nuclear: evidence for activation of peroxisome proliferator-activated receptors Br. J. Pharmacol. (2007). , 152(5), 576-582.

[94] Stella, N, Schweitzer, P, & Piomelli, D. A second endogenous cannabinoid that modulates long-term potentiation Nature (1997). , 388, 773-778.

[95] Beltramo, M, & Piomelli, D. Carrier-mediated transport and enzymatic hydrolysis of the endogenous cannabinoid 2-arachidonylglycerol Neuropharmacology (2000). , 11, 1231-1235.

[96] Di Marzo VTargeting the endocannabinoid system: to enhance or reduce? Nat Rev Drug Discov (2008). , 7, 438-455.

[97] Kozak, K. R, Rowlinson, S. W, & Marnett, L. J. Oxygenation of the endocannabinoid, 2 arachidonylglycerol, to glyceryl prostaglandins by cyclooxygenase-2 J Biol Chem (2000). , 275, 33744-33749.

[98] Blankman, J. L, Simon, G. M, & Cravatt, B. F. A comprehensive profile of brain enzymes that hydrolyze the endocannabinoid 2- arachidonoylglycerol Chem Biol (2007). , 14, 1347-1356.

[99] Dixon, W. E. The pharmacology of cannabis indica Br Med J (1899). , 2, 1354-7.

[100] Bicher, H. I, & Mechoulam, R. Pharmacological effects of two active constituents of marihuana Arch Int Pharmacodyn Ther 196 ;, 172, 24-31.

[101] Kosersky, D. S, Dewey, W. L, & Harris, L. S. Antipyretic, analgesic and anti-infl ammatory effects of delta 9-tetrahydrocannabinol in the rat Eur J Pharmacol (1973). , 24, 1-7.

[102] Costa, B, Colleoni, M, Conti, S, Trovato, A. E, Bianchi, M, Sotgiu, M. L, & Giagnoni, G. Repeated treatment with the synthetic cannabinoid WIN 55,212-2 reduces both hyperalgesia and production of pronociceptive mediators in a rat model of neuropathic pain Br J Pharmacol (2004). , 141(1), 4-8.

[103] Ossipov, M. H, Lopez, Y, Nichols, M. L, Bian, D, & Porreca, F. The loss of antinociceptive efficacy of spinal morphine in rats with nerve ligation injury is prevented by reducing spinal afferent drive.Neurosci Lett (1995). , 199(2), 87-90.

[104] Rashid, M. H, Inoue, M, Toda, K, & Ueda, H. Loss of peripheral morphine analgesia contributes to the reduced effectiveness of systemic morphine in neuropathic pain J Pharmacol Exp Ther. (2004). , 309(1), 380-7.

[105] Guindon, J, & Beaulieu, P. Antihyperalgesic effects of local injections of anandamide, ibuprofen, rofecoxib and their combinations in a model of neuropathic pain Neuropharmacology (2006). , 50, 814-823.

[106] Helyes, Z, Németh, J, Thán, M, Bölcskei, K, Pintér, E, & Szolcsányi, J. Inhibitory effect of anandamide on resiniferatoxin-induced sensory neuropeptide release in vivo and neuropathic hyperalgesia in the rat Life Sci (2003). , 73, 2345-2353.

[107] Costa, B, Siniscalco, D, Trovato, A. E, Comelli, F, Sotgiu, M. L, Colleoni, M, Maione, S, Rossi, F, & Giagnoni, G. AM404, an inhibitor of anandamide uptake, prevents pain

behaviour and modulates cytokine and apoptotic pathways in a rat model of neuropathic pain Br J Pharmacol (2006). , 148, 1022-1032.

[108] Martin, W. J, Coffin, P. O, Attias, E, Balinsky, M, Tsou, K, & Walker, J. M. Anatomical basis for cannabinoid-induced antinociception as revealed by intracerebral microinjections Brain Res. (1999).

[109] Maione, S, Bisogno, T, De Novellis, V, Palazzo, E, Cristino, L, Valenti, M, Petrosino, S, Guglielmotti, V, & Rossi, F. Di Marzo V. Elevation of endocannabinoid levels in the ventrolateral periaqueductal grey through inhibition of fatty acid amide hydrolase affects descending nociceptive pathways via both CB1 and TRPV1 receptors. J Pharmacol Exp Ther (2006). , 316, 969-982.

[110] Racz, I, Nadal, X, Alferink, J, Baños, J. E, Rehnelt, J, Martín, M, Pintado, B, Gutierrez-adan, A, Sanguino, E, Manzanares, J, Zimmer, A, & Maldonado, R. Crucial role of CB(2) cannabinoid receptor in the regulation of central immune responses during neuropathic pain. J Neurosci (2008a). , 28(46), 12125-35.

[111] Racz, I, Nadal, X, Alferink, J, Baños, J. E, Rehnelt, J, Martín, M, Pintado, B, Gutierrez-adan, A, Sanguino, E, Bellora, N, Manzanares, J, & Zimmer, A. Maldonado R Interferon-gamma is a critical modulator of CB(2) cannabinoid receptor signaling during neuropathic pain.J Neurosci. (2008B). , 28(46), 12136-45.

[112] Anand, P, Whiteside, G, Fowler, C. J, & Hohmann, A. G. Targeting CB2 receptors and the endocannabinoid system for the treatment of pain Brain Res Rev (2009). , 60(1), 255-66.

[113] Hampson, R. E, & Deadwyler, S. A. Cannabinoids, hippocampal function and memory. Life Sci (1999). Review

[114] Pertwee, R. G. The central neuropharmacology of psychotropic cannabinoids. Pharmacol Ther. (1988). Review

[115] Maccarrone, M, & Wenger, T. Effects of cannabinoids on hypothalamic and reproductive function. Handb Exp Pharmacol (2005).

[116] Ibrahim, M. M, Lai, J, Vanderah, T. W, Makriyannis, A, & Porreca, F. CB2 cannabinoid receptor agonists: pain relief without psychoactive effects? Curr Opin Pharmacol (2003). Review., 3(1), 62-7.

[117] Maione, S, Piscitelli, F, Gatta, L, Vita, D, De Petrocellis, L, Palazzo, E, & De Novellis, V. Di Marzo V. Non-psychoactive cannabinoids modulate the descending pathway of antinociception in anaesthetized rats through several mechanisms of action Br J Pharmacol (2011). , 162(3), 584-96.

[118] Costa, B, Trovato, A. E, Comelli, F, Giagnoni, G, & Colleoni, M. The non-psychoactive cannabis constituent cannabidiol is an orally effective therapeutic agent in rat chronic inflammatory and neuropathic pain Eur J Pharmacol (2007).

[119] Reid, A. J, Sun, M, Wiberg, M, Downes, S, Terenghi, G, & Kingham, P. J. Nerve repair with adipose-derived stem cells protects dorsal root ganglia neurons from apoptosis. Neuroscience. (2011). , 199, 515-522.

[120] Siniscalco, D, Rossi, F, & Maione, S. Stem cell therapy for neuropathic pain treatment. J Stem Cells and Regenerative Medicine (2008). vol III (1).

[121] Siniscalco, D, Bradstreet, J. J, & Antonucci, N. Cell therapies for Autism Spectrum Disorders. Autism Spectrum Disorders: New Research. (2012). Edited by : Nova Science Publishers, Hauppauge, NY.

[122] Dadon-nachum, M, Sadan, O, Srugo, I, Melamed, E, & Offen, D. Differentiated mesenchymal stem cells for sciatic nerve injury. Stem Cell Rev (2011a). , 7(3), 664-71.

[123] Martínez de Albornoz PDelgado PJ, Forriol F, Maffulli N. Non-surgical therapies for peripheral nerve injury. Br Med Bull (2011). , 100, 73-100.

[124] Dadon-nachum, M, Melamed, E, & Offen, D. Stem cells treatment for sciatic nerve injury. Expert Opin Biol Ther (2011b). , 11(12), 1591-1597.

[125] Azizi, S. A, Stokes, D, & Augelli, B. J. DiGirolamo C, Prockop DJ. Engraftment and migration of human bone marrow stromal cells implanted in the brains of albino rats- similarities to astrocyte grafts. Proc. Natl. Acad. Sci USA(1998). , 95, 3908-3913.

[126] Marconi, S, Castiglione, G, Turano, E, Bissolotti, G, Angiari, S, Farinazzo, A, Constantin, G, Bedogni, G, Bedogni, A, & Bonetti, B. Human adipose-derived mesenchymal stem cells systemically injected promote peripheral nerve regeneration in the mouse model of sciatic crush. Tissue Eng Part A. (2012).

[127] Siniscalco, D. Transplantation of human mesenchymal stem cells in the study of neuropathic pain. Methods Mol Biol. (2010). , 617, 337-345.

[128] Dezawa, M. Future views and challenges to the peripheral nerve regeneration by cell based therapy. Rinsho Shinkeigaku (2005). , 45(11), 877-879.

[129] Frattini, F. Pereira Lopes FR, Almeida FM, Rodrigues RF, Boldrini LC, Tomaz MA, Baptista AF, Melo PA, Martinez AM. Mesenchymal Stem Cells in a Polycaprolactone Conduit Promote Sciatic Nerve Regeneration and Sensory Neuron Survival After Nerve Injury. Tissue Eng Part A. (2012). in press.

[130] Malandrini, A, Eramo, D, Palmeri, C, Gaudiano, S, Gambelli, C, Sicurelli, S, Berti, F, Formichi, G, Kuqo, P, Dotti, A, & Federico, M. T. A. Peripheral neuropathy in late-onset Krabbe disease: report of three cases. Neurol Sci. (2012). in press.

[131] Siddiqi, Z. A, Sanders, D. B, & Massey, J. M. Peripheral neuropathy in Krabbe disease: effect of hematopoietic stem cell transplantation. Neurology. (2006). , 67(2), 268-272.

[132] Kim, H, Kim, J. J, & Yoon, Y. S. Emerging therapy for diabetic neuropathy: cell therapy targeting vessels and nerves. Endocr Metab Immune Disord Drug Targets. (2012). , 12(2), 168-178.

[133] Naruse, K, Sato, J, Funakubo, M, Hata, M, Nakamura, N, Kobayashi, Y, Kamiya, H, Shibata, T, Kondo, M, Himeno, T, Matsubara, T, Oiso, Y, & Nakamura, J. Transplantation of bone marrow-derived mononuclear cells improves mechanical hyperalgesia, cold allodynia and nerve function in diabetic neuropathy. PLoS One (2011). e27458.

[134] Ebben, J. D, Zorniak, M, Clark, P. A, & Kuo, J. S. Introduction to induced pluripotent stem cells: advancing the potential for personalized medicine. World Neurosurg (2011).

[135] Uemura, T, Takamatsu, K, Ikeda, M, Okada, M, Kazuki, K, Ikada, Y, & Nakamura, H. Transplantation of induced pluripotent stem cell-derived neurospheres for peripheral nerve repair. Biochem Biophys Res Commun (2012). , 419(1), 130-135.

[136] Walsh, S. K, Kumar, R, Grochmal, J. K, Kemp, S. W, Forden, J, & Midha, R. Fate of stem cell transplants in peripheral nerves. Stem Cell Res. (2012). , 8(2), 226-238.

[137] Ren, Z, Wang, Y, Peng, J, Zhao, Q, & Lu, S. Role of stem cells in the regeneration and repair of peripheral nerves. Rev Neurosci. (2012). , 23(2), 135-143.

[138] Walsh, S, Biernaskie, J, Kemp, S. W, & Midha, R. Supplementation of acellular nerve grafts with skin derived precursor cells promotes peripheral nerve regeneration. Neuroscience (2009). , 164(3), 1097-1107.

[139] Amoh, Y, & Hoffman, R. M. Isolation and culture of hair follicle pluripotent stem (hfPS) cells and their use for nerve and spinal cord regeneration. Methods Mol Biol. (2010). , 585, 401-420.

[140] Amoh, Y, Aki, R, Hamada, Y, Niiyama, S, Eshima, K, Kawahara, K, Sato, Y, Tani, Y, Hoffman, R. M, & Katsuoka, K. Nestin-positive hair follicle pluripotent stem cells can promote regeneration of impinged peripheral nerve injury. J Dermatol. (2012). , 39(1), 33-38.

[141] Hoffman, R. M. The potential of nestin-expressing hair follicle stem cells in regenerative medicine. Expert Opin Biol Ther. (2007). , 7(3), 289-291.

[142] Peng, J, Wang, Y, Zhang, L, Zhao, B, Zhao, Z, Chen, J, Guo, Q, Liu, S, Sui, X, Xu, W, & Lu, S. Human umbilical cord Wharton's jelly-derived mesenchymal stem cells differentiate into a Schwann-cell phenotype and promote neurite outgrowth in vitro. Brain Res Bull. (2011). , 84(3), 235-243.

[143] Sheu, M. L, Cheng, F. C, Su, H. L, Chen, Y. J, Chen, C. J, Chiang, C. M, Chiu, W. T, Sheehan, J, & Pan, H. C. Recruitment by SDF-1α of CD34-positive cells involved in sciatic nerve regeneration. J Neurosurg (2012). , 116(2), 432-444.

[144] Yang, D. Y, Sheu, M. L, Su, H. L, Cheng, F. C, Chen, Y. J, Chen, C. J, Chiu, W. T, Yiin, J. J, Sheehan, J, & Pan, H. C. Dual regeneration of muscle and nerve by intravenous administration of human amniotic fluid-derived mesenchymal stem cells regulated by stromal cell-derived factor-1α in a sciatic nerve injury model. J Neurosurg. (2012). , 116(6), 1357-1367.

[145] Pan, H. C, Cheng, F. C, Chen, C. J, Lai, S. Z, Lee, C. W, Yang, D. Y, Chang, M. H, & Ho, S. P. Post-injury regeneration in rat sciatic nerve facilitated by neurotrophic factors secreted by amniotic fluid mesenchymal stem cells. J Clin Neurosci. (2007). , 14(11), 1089-1098.

[146] Pan, H. C, Yang, D. Y, Ho, S. P, Sheu, M. L, Chen, C. J, Hwang, S. M, Chang, M. H, & Cheng, F. C. Escalated regeneration in sciatic nerve crush injury by the combined therapy of human amniotic fluid mesenchymal stem cells and fermented soybean extracts, Natto. J Biomed Sci. (2009). a..

[147] Pan, H. C, Chen, C. J, Cheng, F. C, Ho, S. P, Liu, M. J, Hwang, S. M, Chang, M. H, & Wang, Y. C. Combination of G-CSF administration and human amniotic fluid mesenchymal stem cell transplantation promotes peripheral nerve regeneration. Neurochem Res. (2009). b., 34(3), 518-527.

[148] Mohseny AB Hogendoorn PCConcise review: Mesenchymal tumors when stem cells go mad. Stem Cells. (2011). , 29, 397-403.

[149] Mahdi-rogers, M, Kazmi, M, Ferner, R, Hughes, R. A, Renaud, S, Steck, A. J, Fuhr, P, Halter, J, Gratwohl, A, & Tyndall, A. Autologous peripheral blood stem cell transplantation for chronic acquired demyelinating neuropathy. J Peripher Nerv Syst (2009). , 14(2), 118-124.

[150] Amato, A. A, Barohn, R. J, Sahenk, Z, Tutschka, P. J, & Mendell, J. R. Polyneuropathy complicating bone marrow and solid organ transplantation. Neurology (1993). , 43, 1513-1518.

[151] Doi, Y, Sugahara, H, Yamamoto, K, Uji-ie, H, Kakimoto, T, & Sakoda, H. Immune-mediated peripheral neuropathy occurring simultaneously with recurrent graft-versus-host disease after allogenic hematopoietic stem cell transplantation. Leuk Res. (2012). e, 63-65.

[152] Boiron, J. M, Ellie, E, Vital, A, Marit, G, Rème, T, Vital, C, Broustet, A, & Reiffers, J. Peripheral neuropathy after autologous blood stem cell transplantation for multiple myeloma. Leukemia (1994). , 8(2), 322-326.

[153] Siniscalco, D, Giordano, A, & Galderisi, U. Novel insights in basic and applied stem cell therapy. J Cell Physiol (2012). , 227(5), 2283-2286.

Section 2

Evaluation and Management of Peripheral Neuropathy

Chapter 4

Compression Neuropathies

Javier López Mendoza and
Alexandro Aguilera Salgado

Additional information is available at the end of the chapter

http://dx.doi.org/10.5772/55316

1. Introduction

Upper extremity compression neuropathies are among the most common disorders in plastic surgery, especially in patients with predisposing occupations or with certain medical disorders. In the past two decades a notable increase in the incidence of this entity has occurred. Therefore, it is mandatory to achieve a prompt diagnosis because they can produce important motor and sensory deficiencies that need to be treated before the development of complications, since, despite the capacity for regeneration bestowed on the peripheral nervous system, functions lost as a result of denervation are never fully restored.

2. Etiology

There are many different situations that may be a direct cause of nerve compression. Anatomically, nerves can be compressed when traversing fibro-osseous tunnels, passing between muscle layers, through traction as they cross joints or buckling during certain movements of the wrist and elbow. Other causes include trauma, direct pressure and space-occupying lesions at any level in the upper extremity.

There are other situations that are not a direct cause of nerve compression, but may increase the risk and may predispose the nerve to be compressed specially when the soft tissues are swollen like synovitis, pregnancy, hypothyroidism, diabetes or alcoholism [1].

Physicians in touch with patients who suffer from upper extremity compression neuropathies must apply all of their skills to correctly distinguish symptomatic nerve entrapment form other neurologic entities such as myelopathy, braquial plexopathy, radiculopathy, and other central nervous system disorders, that can mimic peripheral nerve entrapment.

Besides these pathologies, the differential diagnosis must include painful rheumatologic and orthopedic disorders; and other psychological entities, such as somatoform and factitious disorders.

3. Pathophysiology

When nerve fibers undergo compression, the response depends on the force applied at the site and the duration. Acute, brief compression results in a focal conduction block as a result of local ischemia, being reversible if the duration of compression is transient. On the other hand, if the focal compression is prolonged, ischemic changes appear, followed by endoneurial edema and secondary perineurial thickening. These histological alterations will aggravate the changes in the microneural circulation and will increase the sensitivity of the neuron sheath to ischemia. If the compression continues, we will find focal demyelination, which typically results in a greater involvement of motor than sensory nerve fibers. Even at this point clinical and electrophysiologic signs can resolve within a period of weeks to months.

As the duration of compression increases beyond several hours, more diffuse demyelination will appear, being the last event an injury to the axons themselves. This process begins at the distal end of compression or injury, a process termed wallerian degeneration. These neural changes may not appear at a uniform fashion among the whole neural sheath depending on the distribution of the compressive forces, causing mixed demyelinating and axonal injury resulting from a combination of mechanical distortion of the nerve, ischemic injury, and impaired axonal flow [2].

4. Clinical evaluation

4.1. History

We must begin with a complete history of the patient, asking about preexisting diseases that may be a direct cause of the neuropathy or may exacerbate it like diabetes, hypothyroidism, alcoholism, rheumatologic or orthopedic problems and any history of trauma or surgeries that may explain his or her symptoms.

The symptoms we may find in our patients will depend on diverse factors, mainly in the nature of the nerve involved, if it is primary motor, sensitive or both, and the anatomic location of the site of compression. The principal affections we will find will be hypoesthesia of the territory of the sensitive nerve or a complete anesthesia in more chronic conditions. In case of motor nerve compression, symptoms will be related to a progressive loss of function to a complete muscular atrophy in severe cases.

We need to investigate when did the symptoms began, if they were progressive or sudden, which movements are limited or impaired, if hypoesthesia or complete loss of sensation is present, accompanying symptoms, and if they have improved with time or with a particular action taken by the patient.

4.2. Physical exam

Besides a complete history of our patient, a thorough nerve exam needs to be addressed based on the knowledge of the upper extremity nerves anatomy in order to determine the possible site of compression. Our physical exam must include a sensitive and a motor evaluation of the complete upper extremity, beginning with the evaluation of specific movements of the shoulder, arm, forearm, elbow, wrist and digits to determine which muscles are affected and the range of motion of each of these muscles. Next, the sensitivity must be tested, light touch, pain, pressure, vibration and two-point discrimination among the specific distribution of the main nerve involved. There are some complementary tests we may apply in order to guide our exam according to the nerve we think is involved. These specific tests will be discussed further in the chapter [3].

5. Electrophysiology

Electrophysiologic testing is part of the evaluation, but it never substitutes a complete history and a thorough physical examination. These tests can detect physiologic abnormalities in the course of motor and sensory axons. There are two main electrophysiologic tests: needle electromyography and nerve conduction, which permit differentiating between a focal mononeuropathy, a radiculopathy, and a plexopathy, or the discovery of a more diffuse process, such as a systemic peripheral neuropathy or motor neuron disorder.

The electromyography detects the voluntary or spontaneous generated electrical activity. The registry of this activity is made through the needle insertion, at rest and during muscular activity to assess duration, amplitude, configuration and recruitment after injury. Recruitment will be affected if demyelination occurs, but will not result in abnormal spontaneous activity. Meanwhile, axonal injury will result in both recruitment and abnormal spontaneous activity, which will not be seen on needle electromyography until 2 weeks after the initial insult [4].

Nerve conduction assesses for both sensory and motor nerves. This study consists in applying a voltage simulator to the skin over different points of the nerve in order to record the muscular action potential, analyzing the amplitude, duration, area, latency and conduction velocity. The amplitude indicates the number of available nerve fibers. Some authors consider diminished amplitude below 50% to be suggestive of compression. In such cases, we will find a normal response to distal stimulation but no response proximal to the site of entrapment. If the compression progresses, our results will be compatible with axonal degeneration with diminished amplitude of the response with relative preservation of the conduction velocity and distal latency until the remaining axons are completely damaged [5].

6. Median nerve

6.1. Anatomy

The median nerve is formed in the axilla by a branch each from the medial and lateral chords of the brachial plexus, receiving fibers from C6, C7, C8 and T1 roots. It arises anterior to the axillary artery, descending distally through the arm lateral to the brachial artery till it reaches the medial aspect of the arm. It is important to know that the median nerve has no branches above the cubital fossa. It enters the cubital fossa lateral to the brachialis tendon passing between the two heads of the pronator teres giving off the anterior interosseus branch (Figure 1).

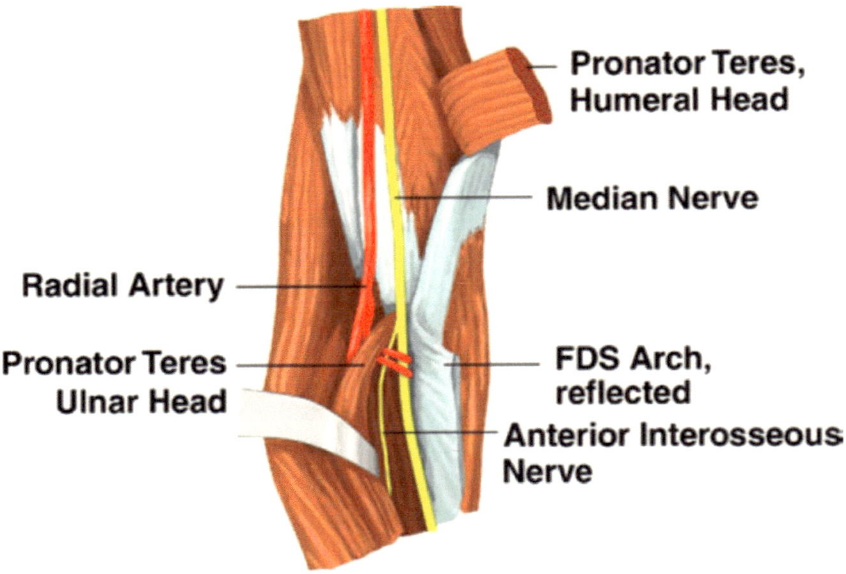

Figure 1. Median nerve descending lateral to brachial artery, giving off the anterior interosseus branch between the two heads of the pronator teres.

The nerve continues in the forearm between the flexor digitorium profundus and flexor digitorium superficialis, giving off above the wrist the palmar cutaneous branch that supplies the skin of the central portion of the palm. In the forearm it supplies the pronator teres, flexor carpi radialis, flexor digitorium superficialis and profundus, flexor pollicis longus and pronator quadratus [6] (Figure 2).

http://dx.doi.org/10.5772/55316

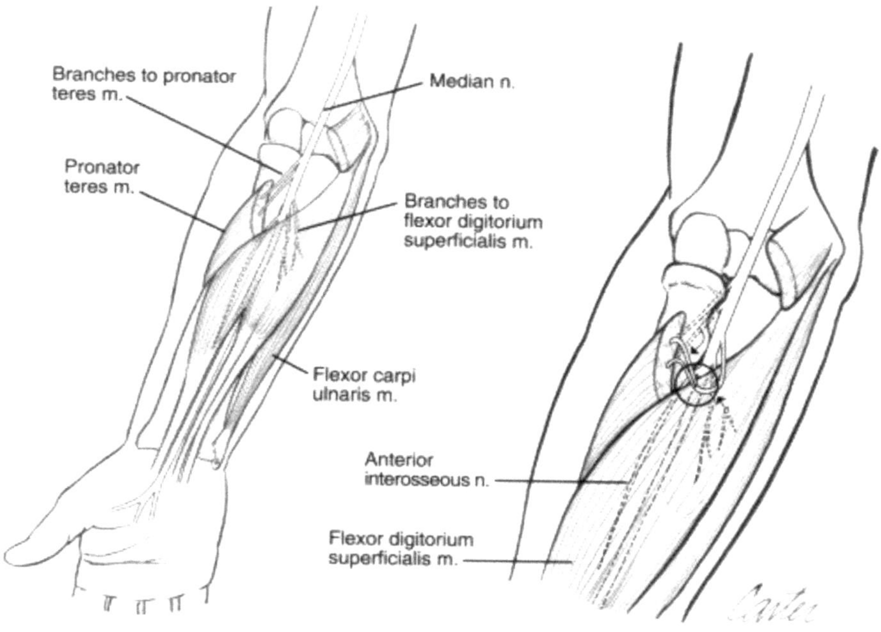

Figure 2. Branches and supplied muscles by the median nerve in the forearm.

Finally, it enters the hand through the carpal tunnel, running beneath the transverse carpal ligament, superficial to nine tendons: four of the flexor digitorium superficialis, four of the flexor digitorium profundus and one of the flexor pollicis longus. Distally it supplies the thenar eminence muscles and the lateral two lumbricalis, providing sensation to the first 3 digits and the lateral aspect of the fourth digit. (Figure 3).

6.2. Median nerve entrapment

There are three well-described entrapment syndromes involving the median nerve or its branches, namely pronator teres syndrome, anterior interosseous syndrome and carpal tunnel syndrome according to the level of entrapment. Each one of these syndromes presents with different clinical signs and symptoms, electrophysiologic results and requires different techniques for their release.

6.3. Pronator teres syndrome (Proximal compression)

6.3.1. Sites of compression

This is the most proximal compression site of the median nerve. It is due to compression of the median nerve as it passes through pronator teres. It may also be compressed upon the lacertus fibrosus (fascial sheet attached to biceps tendon), at the arched origin of the flexor digitorium superficialis or at the ligament of Struthers (connects medial epicondyle with a supracondylar process of humerus).

6.3.2. Diagnosis

The onset is insidious and is suggested when the early sensory disturbances are greater on the thumb and index finger, mainly tingling, numbness and dysaesthesia in the median nerve distribution. Patients will also complain of increased pain in the proximal forearm and greater hand numbness with sustained power gripping or rotation because these movements tighten the fibrous origin of the superficial flexor muscles beneath which the median nerve passes. There is no nocturnal preference.

In the physical exam we may find a positive Tinel's sign at site of proximal compression within the antecubital fossa, negative over the carpal tunnel. Phalen's test will be negative. Generally, the neurophysiological exam will be normal, although in severe cases we may find fibrillations and sharp positive spikes in pronator quadratus and flexor pollicis longus.

6.3.3. Treatment

Surgical decompression is the definitive treatment. The incision should be distal to the elbow, oblique and parallel to the proximal margin of the pronator teres muscle, followed by an external neurolysis of the nerve performed proximally between the two heads of the pronator teres, and distally as it passes beneath the flexor digitorium superficialis muscle.

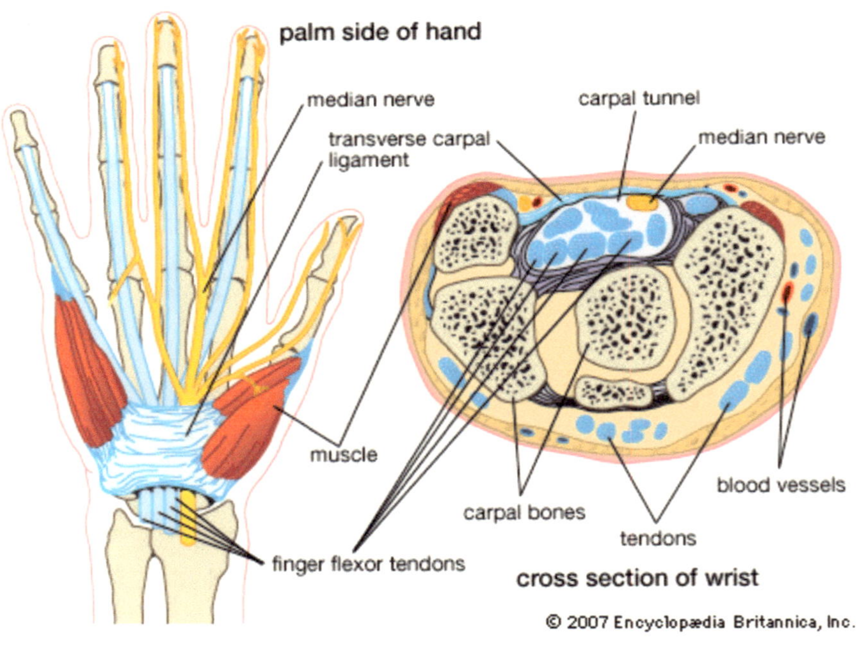

Figure 3. Carpal tunnel limits and branches of the median nerve in the hand.

http://dx.doi.org/10.5772/55316

6.4. Anterior interosseous syndrome

6.4.1. Innervation

The anterior interosseous nerve classically innervates these muscles: flexor pollicis longus, pronator quadratus and the radial half of flexor digitorium profundus. These muscles are in the deep level of the anterior compartment of the forearm.

6.4.2. Causes of compression

The most common cause of this syndrome is a spontaneous fracture, probably due to brachial neuritis. Other causes include a space-occupying lesion, open fractures, elbow dislocation, compartment syndrome affecting the flexor compartment of the forearm, compression by the deep head of the pronator teres, the arch of flexor digitorium superficialis, or by Gantzer's muscle (accessory head of flexor pollicis longus).

6.4.3. Diagnosis

It presents principally as weakness of the index finger and thumb, and the patient may complain of diffuse pain in the proximal forearm, which may be exacerbated during exercise and diminished with rest. The vast majority of patients begin with pain in the upper arm, elbow and forearm, often preceding the motor symptoms. Pain is a common feature of anterior interosseus nerve compression, but it is not a predictive sign for differentiating an inflammatory from a mechanical origin.

During physical exam, the patient will be unable to bend the tip of the thumb and tip of index finger. The typical symptom is the inability to form an "O" with the thumb and index finger. Since flexor pollicis longus and flexor digitorium profundus to the index and middle finger are paralyzed, the patient will not be able to flex the interphalangeal joint of the thumb and the distal interphalangeal joint of the index finger. Sometimes, the motor branches to pronator teres, flexor carpi radialis and/or palmaris longus are also involved. [7] Spinner [8] has described a sign in which upon making a fist, the tips of the index finger and thumb remain conspicuously excluded. The examination of the pronator quadratus is difficult and unreliable. With the elbow bent at 90º, the patient is asked to forcibly pronate the forearm against resistance of the examiner.

The anterior interosseus nerve provides no sensory fibers to the skin, therefore, the sensation and sweating in the median nerve distribution is preserved. Abnormal sensibility in the median nerve distribution in the presence of an anterior interosseus syndrome, suggests a proximal median compression neuropathy involving fascicles of the anterior interosseus nerve. [9]

Electrophysiologic tests may reveal denervation and weakness of the muscles innervated by the anterior interosseous nerve. Other studies like an MRI should be necessary in order to discard space-occupying lesions and the involvement of bone and other structures.

6.4.4. Treatment

If the onset was spontaneous and there is no evident lesion on MRI, supportive care and corticosteroid injections with observation for 4 to 6 weeks is usually accepted management. The degree of recovery is unpredictable. If the symptoms continue we may continue with a surgical treatment where a detachment or resection of the deep head of the pronator teres muscle is performed. If there is no evident recovery, we may have to consider tendon transfers.

6.5. Carpal tunnel syndrome

This is the most frequently encountered compression neuropathy in the upper limb. It is a mechanical compression of the median nerve through the fixed space of the rigid carpal tunnel. The incidence in the United States has been estimated at 1 to 3 cases per 1,000 subjects per year, with a prevalence of 50 cases per 1,000 subjects per year. [10] It is more common in women than in men (2:1), perhaps because the carpal tunnel itself may be smaller in women than in men. The dominant hand is usually affected first and produces the most severe pain. It usually occurs in adults, being the peak age range for development 45 to 60 years, and only 10% of patients are younger than 30 years. The risk of developing carpal tunnel syndrome is not confined to people in a single industry or job, but it is especially common in those performing assembly line work, manufacturing, sewing, cleaning and poultry or fish packing.

6.5.1. Anatomy

The carpal tunnel runs beneath the transverse carpal ligament, which transversely connects the pisiform, hamate, scaphoid and trapezium and longitudinally connects the deep fascia of the forearm and the palmar fascia. It contains the median nerve, 9 tendons previously described and the motor branch of the median nerve. There are three major patterns of branching of the recurrent motor branch: extraligamentous (50%), subligamentous (31%) and transligamentous (23%) [11].

6.5.2. Carpal tunnel pressure

The lowest carpal tunnel pressure at rest with wrist in neutral position is 2.5mmHg. In full wrist flexion it normally rises up to 30mmHg. In patients with carpal tunnel syndrome, this pressure rises to 30mmHg and 90mmHg respectively (Phalen's test provokes this rise in pressure).

6.5.3. Etiology

There is still some controversy among the activities that may be a direct cause of carpal tunnel syndrome. It is believed to be idiopathic in the majority of cases and it has been related to repetitive prolonged wrist extension causing mechanical irritation, synovitis and eventually compressive neuropathy of the median nerve. Trauma can be another cause of this syndrome mainly among 5% of wrist fractures and 60% of lunate dislocations. Other rare disorders include renal failure and haemodialysis, hypothyroidism, pregnancy and some space-occupying lesions like ganglions and nerve tumours.

http://dx.doi.org/10.5772/55316

6.6. Anomalous interconnections

In some cases we may find these anomalous interconnections that may explain some clinical findings not attributable to the median nerve like little finger numbness in carpal tunnel syndrome:

- **Martin Gruber**: Motor interconnections from median to ulnar nerve in forearm.
- **Richie-Cannieu**: Motor and sensory interconnections from median to ulnar nerve in the hand.

6.6.1. Diagnosis

It is mainly clinic, but complementary electrophysiologic tests should be ordered. It is typically first manifested by numbness, discomfort and parestesias of the thumb, index finger, middle finger and the radial side of the ring finger. As the symptoms progress, the patient may be awakened from sleep, referring constant numbness and pain. Pain may develop on the anterior wrist or at distal forearm at the carpal tunnel entrance (Durkin sign) and may be aggravated by elevation of the hand. Skin sensibility is not disturbed in the distribution of the palmar cutaneous branch as this branch is subcutaneous and does not pass through the carpal tunnel. Phalen and Tinel tests are highly reliable for diagnosis of carpal tunnel syndrome. If both tests are positive, there is a 91% chance of an accurate diagnosis. In advanced stages of carpal tunnel syndrome we may find thenar atrophy, which is associated with axonal damage [12].

Graham et al, developed a list of 6 clinical criteria (CTS-6) for the diagnosis of carpal tunnel syndrome, having all of them a statistically significant probability of being associated with this entity [13] (Table 1).

Electrodiagnostic studies are reliable for evaluation of suspected carpal tunnel syndrome, but in questionable cases, clinical evaluation supersedes these studies. Abnormalities on electrophysiologic testing, in association with specific symptoms and signs, are considered the criterion standard for carpal tunnel syndrome diagnosis. Electrophysiologic testing also can provide an accurate assessment of how severe the damage to the nerve is, thereby directing management and providing objective criteria for the determination of prognosis. Carpal tunnel syndrome is usually divided into mild, moderate and severe. In general, patients with mild carpal tunnel syndrome have sensory abnormalities alone on electrophysiologic testing, and patients with sensory plus motor abnormalities have moderate carpal tunnel syndrome. However, any evidence of axonal loss is classified as severe carpal tunnel syndrome. [14]. Electromyography shows fibrillation and positive sharp spikes in severe compression with muscle atrophy. Nerve conduction may reveal an increase in terminal sensory latency, sensory conduction velocity or motor conduction velocity when compared with the other hand.

No imaging studies are considered routine in the diagnosis of carpal tunnel syndrome. Magnetic resonance imaging of the carpal tunnel is particularly useful preoperatively if a space-occupying lesion in the carpal tunnel is suggested. MRI does not rule out the multitude of other differential diagnoses and it is time consuming and resource intensive. [15] The same thing occurs with the use of ultrasound in the diagnosis of this entity, because there can be problems differentiating the median nerve from surrounding soft tissue, and some studies report that it does not correlate well with both clinical and electrodiagnostic criteria, limiting its role in diagnosis. [16]

CTS-6. Diagnostic Clinical Criteria for Carpal Tunnel Syndrome
1: Numbness and tingling in the median nerve distribution
2: Nocturnal numbness
3: Weakness and/or atrophy of the thenar musculature
4: Tinel's sign
5: Phalen's test
6: Loss of 2-point discrimination

Table 1. Diagnostic Clinical Criteria for Carpal Tunnel Syndrome

6.6.2. Treatment

It can be divided in non-operative and surgical decompression of the carpal tunnel. The non-operative treatment is based in splintage of the wrist in a neutral position for three weeks and steroid injections. This therapy has variable results, with a success rate up to 76% during one year, but with a recurrence rate as high as 94%. Non-operative treatment is indicated in patients with intermittent symptoms, initial stages and during pregnancy [17].

The only definitive treatment for carpal tunnel syndrome is surgical expansion of the carpal tunnel by transection of the transverse carpal ligament. There is much controversy over what is the most appropriate surgical technique for decompression of the carpal tunnel, either by and open or by an endoscopic approach. In an attempt to resolve this issue, numerous prospective randomized trials have been reported comparing both techniques in terms of safety, efficacy, perioperative morbidity, relative costs and the return to preoperative functional status with variable results. One of the latest studies regarding this matter, was a systematic review performed in 2007 by Sholten et al, published by the Cochrane Collaboration that compared both techniques, reporting equal outcome scores by three months and with rates of complications similar in most studies, concluding there is no strong evidence to support the need for conversion from open techniques to endoscopic or more limited techniques. In addition, some other authors like Atroshi and Trumble have similar conclusions, reporting that both techniques appear to be safe and effective methods of treating carpal tunnel syndrome with no clear long-term differences in outcomes measures to support one method as clearly superior to the other. The decision as to which procedure is most appropriate, therefore, remains a matter of choice for surgeons and patients [18,19].

Other approaches like neurolysis of median nerve have been studied. Mackinnon found that it is not beneficial, with recurrence of symptoms because of internal wound healing. It would just be indicated in patients with thenar atrophy, loss of sensation or the presence of a neuroma. [20] Likewise, synovectomy is just indicated in cases of severe thenosynovytis resulting from rheumatoid arthritis, amyloidosis or renal failure. [21]

6.6.3. Complications

Some of the complications reported can be complex regional pain syndrome, scar pain, pillar pain, infection, injury to the palmar cutaneous branch or to the motor branch of the median nerve, vascular or tendon injury, and recurrence reported in 1% or less of the patients.

7. Ulnar nerve

7.1. Anatomy

The ulnar nerve contains fibers from C8 and T1 and is the largest terminal branch of the medial cord of the brachial plexus. The nerve enters the arm with the axillary artery and courses medially to the brachial artery before piercing the intermuscular septum approaching the elbow. It then travels along the border of the medial head of the triceps and enters the postcondylar groove lateral to the medial epicondyle [22]. At the elbow, the ulnar nerve enters the forearm between the medial epicondyle and the olecranon through the cubital tunnel. The roof of the cubital tunnel is a fibrous aponeurosis that thickens to form the cubital tunnel retinaculum or arcuate ligament of Osborne. This retinaculum connects the tendinous origin of the humeral and ulnar heads of the flexor carpi ulnaris, giving off branches to the elbow joint [23] (Figure 4).

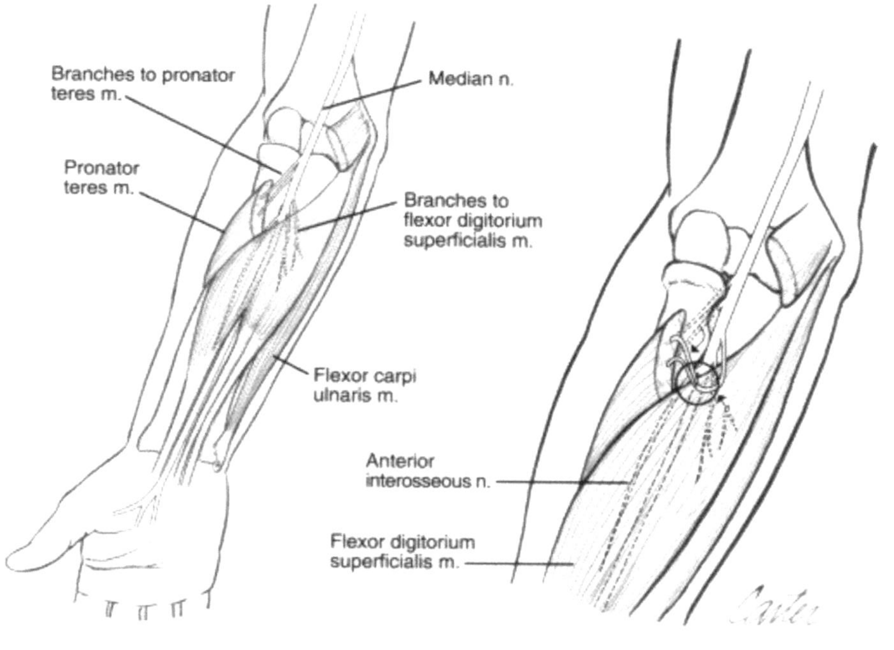

Figure 4. Ulnar nerve anatomy at the elbow.

Exiting the tunnel, the ulnar nerve pierces the flexor pronator aponeurosis, innervating the flexor digitorum muscles before entering Guyon's canal at the wrist. The terminal branches of the ulnar nerve supply motor innervation to the adductor pollicis, the flexor pollicis brevis, the hypothenar muscles, the third and fourth lumbricalis, and all of the interosseous muscles. The sensory distribution of the nerve includes the palmar and dorsal medial aspects of the hand, often including half of the ring finger (Figure 5).

7.2. Ulnar nerve entrapment

The ulnar nerve, like the median nerve, is susceptible to compression neuropathies at proximal and distal levels. Proximally, the most common site of compression is the cubital tunnel as the ulnar nerve enters the forearm between the medial epicondyle and the olecranon. Other potential sites of compression at the elbow, are between the humeral and ulnar heads of the flexor carpi ulnaris muscle and 3cm distal to the cubital tunnel, when the ulnar nerve pierces the flexor pronator aponeurosis. Distally, the ulnar nerve can be compressed at the Guyon's canal at the wrist. Each one of these sites of compression present with different signs and symptoms which will be described next.

7.3. Cubital tunnel syndrome (Ulnar nerve compression at the elbow)

7.3.1. Etiology

The majority of cases occur spontaneously with no documented history of trauma, caused by adhesions that prevent the nerve's gliding with elbow flexion, stretching the nerve behind the epicondyle that impairs nerve conduction. Other causes include direct pressure either by tumors, external swelling-synovium, lipomas or osteophytes, subluxation over the medial epicondyle or just by inadequate space in the cubital tunnel and over the potential sites of compression mentioned above [24].

7.3.2. Diagnosis

The patient may present both motor and sensory disturbances, including pain at the medial portion of the proximal third of the forearm, parestesias or anesthesia of palmar and dorsal surfaces of the ring and small fingers, and ulnar innervated intrinsic muscles weakness, which can present atrophy in late stages. During physical exam, the acute flexion of the elbow for 30 seconds usually accentuates the sensory symptoms and also may cause tingling in the little and ring finger, promptly relieved by extending the elbow. A positive Tinel's sign at the posterior elbow will be referred to the small finger.

We may also find a positive Froment's sign and a positive Wartenburg's sign (Figure 6). Froment's sign tests for the action of adductor pollicis, which is weak with an ulnar nerve compression. A patient is asked to hold an object, usually a flat object such as a piece of paper, between their thumb and index finger. The examines then attempts to pull the object out of the patient's hands. A normal individual will be able to maintain a hold on the object without difficulty. With ulnar nerve palsy, the patient will experience difficulty maintaining a hold and

http://dx.doi.org/10.5772/55316

will compensate by flexing the flexor pollicis longus of the thumb to maintain grip pressure. Clinically, this compensation manifests as flexion of the interphalangeal joint of the thumb.

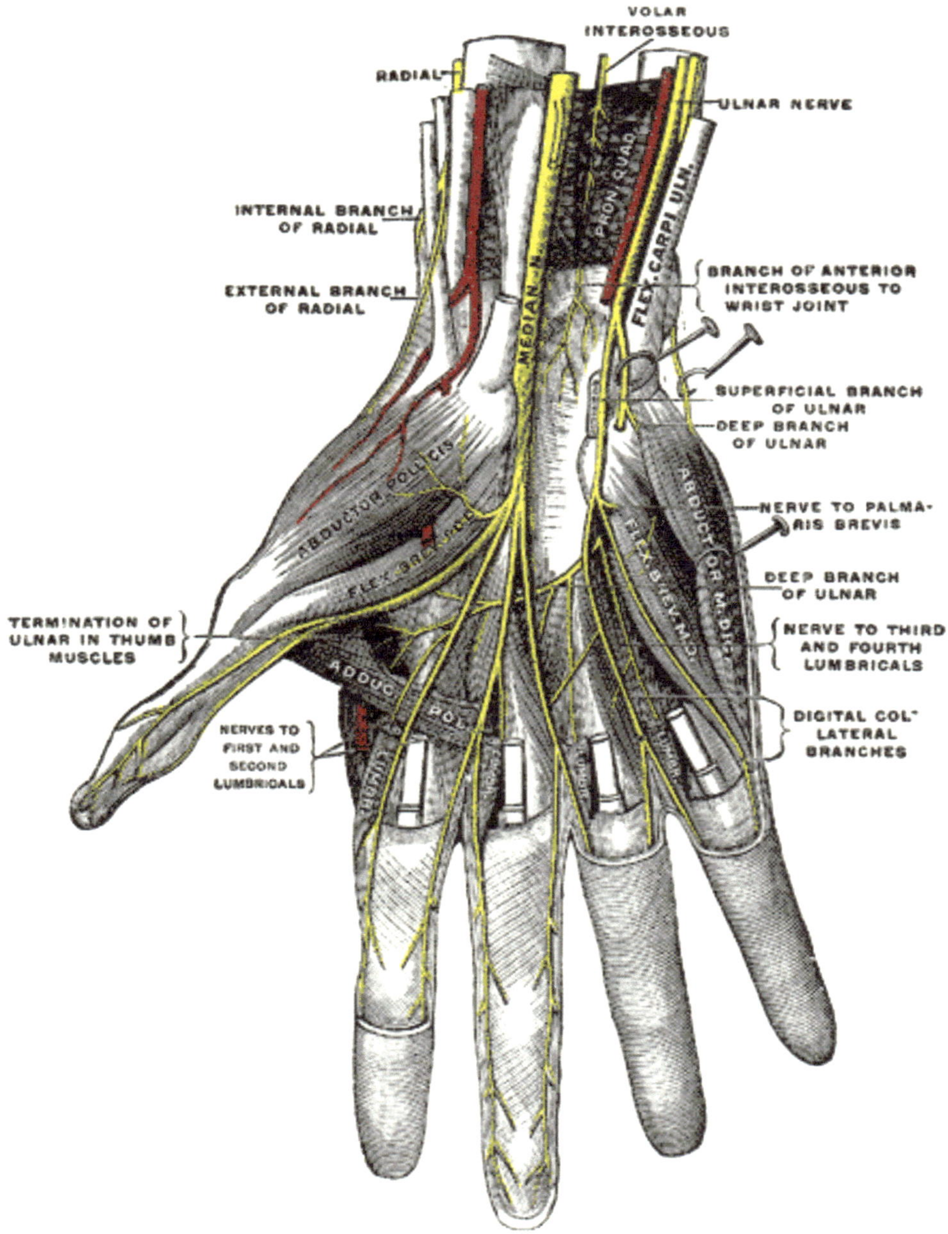

Figure 5. Ulnar nerve anatomy in the hand.

Simultaneous hyperextension of the thumb metacarpophalangeal joint is indicative of ulnar nerve compromise.

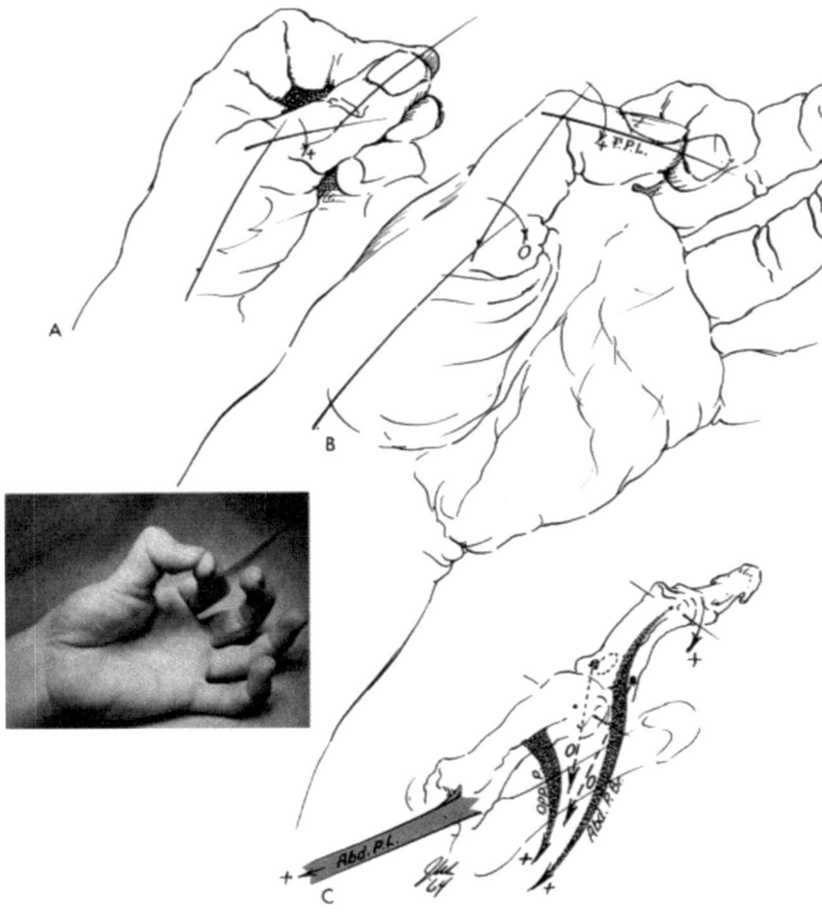

Figure 6. Positive Froment's sign.

On the other hand we have Wartenburg's sign. The patient is placed with wrist in neutral position and forearm fully pronated and instructed to perform full extension of all the fingers. Once digits are extended, patient is asked to fully abduct all fingers and then adduct all fingers. A positive signs is indicated with the observation of abduction of the 5th digit, with inability to adduct the 5th finger when extended. The inability to perform adducted digital extension is due to weakness in ulnar innervated intrinsic muscles.

Electromyography and nerve conduction may reveal a drop in speed conduction or alterations in the sensitive latency, but these studies may be normal, specially in postural conditions, requiring complementary studies like X-rays or an MRI if a space occupying lesion is suspected or if there is a conduction block with established compression but the site is not clear.

http://dx.doi.org/10.5772/55316

7.3.3. Treatment

It is divided in non-operative and operative options. The non-operative treatment is advised in patients with mainly postural symptoms by avoiding flexing the elbow or leaning on the inner side of the elbow, and by splinting the elbow at 45º extension at night, changing the patient's sleeping posture. One may consider surgery in more advanced stages, if the patient refers numbness or weakness in the hand, which may represent axonal demyelination and muscle atrophy.

Surgical management of the ulnar nerve entrapment at the elbow is determined by the patient's preoperative symptoms and intraoperative findings. It includes transposition of the nerve anterior to the axis of rotation of the elbow so that elbow flexion relaxes rather than stretches the nerve. Commonly performed procedures include simple decompression by unroofing the cubital tunnel, anterior subcutaneous transposition, intramuscular transposition, submuscular transposition, and medial epicondylectomy.

In selected cases, simple decompression of the cubital tunnel and the anterior subcutaneous transposition may be effective, but the ulnar nerve may be more susceptible to trauma injuries as it becomes more superficial. The submuscular anterior transposition is the best operation for cubital tunnel syndrome when an adequate distal mobilization is performed. Other options include a percutaneous and endoscopic release being both technically possible but not generally recommended because of poor results and a high incidence of recurrence [25].

7.3.4. Complications

Complications are rare but they include haematoma, infection, neuroma, damage to medial cutaneous nerve of forearm and devascularization of the ulnar nerve, which is the worst of the complications.

7.4. Ulnar nerve compression at the wrist

7.4.1. Guyon's canal

At the wrist, the ulnar nerve and artery enter Guyon's canal, which is a fibro-osseous tunnel formed between the pisiform and hamate hook. The floor of the canal is formed by the pisohamate ligamento and the flexor retinaculum, and the roof is the palmaris brevis and the superficial volar carpal ligament (continuation of distal forearm fascia).

Within Guyon's canal, the ulnar nerve bifurcates into superficial and deep branches giving off sensory and motor branches, which innervate intrinsic muscles of the hand previously described in this chapter (Figure 7).

7.4.2. Zones of nerve

As the ulnar nerve enters the wrist through Guyon's canal, it is divided in 3 zones:

i. Proximal to bifurcation of nerve into deep and superficial branches.

ii. Around deep motor branch.

iii. Around superficial sensory branch.

7.4.3. Etiology

The most common cause of Guyon's canal entrapment is a carpal ganglion. The next most common etiology is repeated trauma to the hypothenar area usually related to occupation. Finally, other less frequent causes include osteophytes from pisotriquetral joint, fracture of the hook of hamate, and pseudoaneurysms of the ulnar artery.

7.4.4. Diagnosis

The patient will present with some similar symptoms as in the cubital tunnel syndrome, with some specific differences. In low ulnar neuropathy, the symptoms will not be related to position of the elbow. Also, the sensation at the dorsal aspect of the ulnar border will be preserved, as the dorsal sensory branch of the ulnar nerve has taken off 5 to 10cm proximal to Guyon's canal. The function of flexor carpi ulnaris and flexor digitorium profundus muscles will be preserved. The motor affection will be exclusive of the intrinsic muscles of the hand, which can be measured with lateral pinch between thumb and side of index finger.

The diagnosis is mainly clinic but some other studies may be needed in order to complete our investigation. X-rays are necessary to evaluate the integrity of the osseous components of the canal, ultrasound if we suspect of a ganglion, arteriogram if ulnar artery aneurysm is suspect-

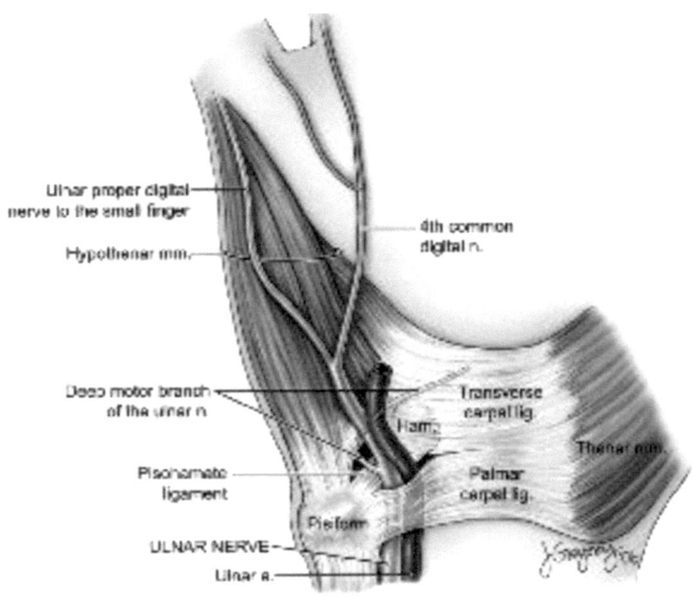

Figure 7. Guyon's canal anatomy.

ed, MRI if precise location of tumours needs to be addressed, and finally electromyography and nerve conduction to confirm the level of conduction block.

7.4.5. Treatment

It consists in surgical decompression of the canal with special care to avoid injury to the dorsal division, which does not pass through the canal. The safest way to decompress the canal is finding the nerve proximal to pisiform and tracing the branches of the nerve distally, progressively unroofing the canal. Once it is open we must treat any pathology we identify like a ganglion or a pseudoaneurysm.

8. Radial nerve

8.1. Anatomy

The radial nerve receives innervation form C5-C8 and T1 roots, being the terminal branch of the posterior cord. It enters the arm behind the brachial artery, medial to the humerus and anterior to the long head of the triceps muscle running through the radial groove at the humerus, giving off branches for both heads of the triceps muscle. It descends distally along the border of the brachialis muscle and approximately 2cm distal to the elbow, the radial nerve divides into the posterior interosseous nerve and the superficial sensory divisions. The posterior interosseous nerve passes beneath the fibrous proximal margin of the supinator muscle, known as the arcade of Frohse, and bifurcates to innervate the extensor carpi ulnaris muscle and the digital extensor muscles. The radial nerve does not innervate any hand muscle [26] (Figure 8).

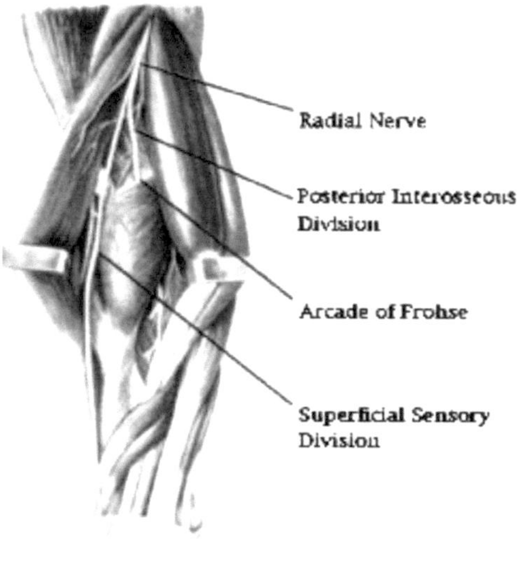

Figure 8. Radial nerve anatomy showing its divisions at the forearm.

8.2. Radial nerve entrapment

Lister et al, in 1979, suggested 4 possible sites of radial nerve compression: the fibrous bands anterior to the radial head, the "radial recurrent fan" of vessels described by Henry, the tendinous margin of the extensor carpi radialis brevis, and the arcade of Frohse. A fifth site of possible compression of this nerve is at the radial tunnel, which represents the fascia at the superficial portion of the supinator muscle that may compress the deep branch of the radial nerve. Nevertheless, the compression of the posterior interosseous branch is the most important entity in this matter (Figure 9).

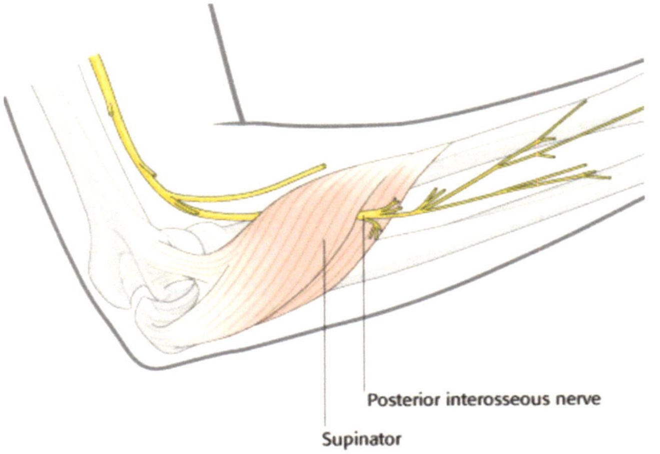

Figure 9. Posterior interosseous branch and its relation with the supinator muscle.

8.3. Proximal radial nerve compression

8.3.1. Etiology

There are many possible causes of proximal radial nerve compression, being the most common by direct pressure in the axilla, traumatic division, iatrogenic injury or by traction. At the elbow, it may be caused by a fibrous band from the shaft of the humerus that crosses the nerve to the lateral epicondyle [27].

8.3.2. Diagnosis

The patient will present with slight weakness of elbow flexion, marked weakness of elbow and wrist extension, finger elevation, thumb retroposition and numbness over the dorsal aspect of thumb base. If the compression is at the elbow, the patient will not have disturbance of the radial wrist extensor muscles as their motor nerves separate from the radial nerve proximal to the elbow, but the sensory branch will be affected as the motor division to the digital extensor muscles. Electrophysiologic studies are not diagnostic unless there is significant denervation.

http://dx.doi.org/10.5772/55316

8.3.3. Treatment

In case of pressure palsy, observation is indicated as most of the symptoms may recover in hours, several weeks or even months. If the patient only presents with moderate symptoms limited to the sensory division of the nerve, a trial of systemic steroids and rest of the arm usually is considered. In severe and progressive cases a surgical decompression may be indicated with a dorsoradial surgical approach [28].

8.4. Posterior interosseous syndrome

8.4.1. Etiology

Brachial neuritis, fibrous bands anterior to the radial head, fibrous proximal edge of extensor carpi radialis brevis, arcade of Frohse, distal edge of supinator, lipomas and synovitis from proximal radioulnar joint or radioocapitellar joint.

8.4.2. Diagnosis

The patient will present with weakness of the hand and wrist often with rapid onset. The wrist extension is preserved but it will move radialwards because of failure of extensor carpi radialis brevis and extensor carpi ulnaris. There will be no elevation of the metacarpophalangeal joints with no retroposition of the thumb. The majority of cases have no sensory disturbance in the distribution of the superficial branch of the radial nerve. Electrophysiologyc studies are of little help; the diagnosis is basically from careful and serial evaluations.

8.4.3. Treatment

The management can be divided in operative and non-operative options. Observation is initially indicated if no space-occupying lesion is suspected up to 12 months. It is accompanied by splinting of the wrist in extension or by the use of a dynamic extension splint. Severe or progressive cases need surgical decompression, which has little risk, very low morbidity, and is typically followed by prompt relief from the pain. The surgery consists in a total external neurolysis of the nerve, starting 2cm distal to the elbow crease carried through the subcutaneous tissues distally.

8.5. Wartenburg's syndrome

8.5.1. Etiology

This syndrome originates from compression of superficial radial nerve as it emerges from beneath brachioradialis muscle to reach the subcutaneous plane over the radial border of the distal forearm. At the point of exit from beneath the muscle, a compression of the nerve can develop. It does not develop spontaneously, but is an infrequent complication of trauma to the midforearm.

8.5.2. Diagnosis

The patient will present local pain and sensory disturbance to the dorsal-lateral skin of the hand, with tingling over back of thumb base, with a positive Tinel's sign at the point of exit of the nerve from beneath the braquiradialis muscle. As this muscle is a supinator muscle pain is accentuated by attempting this motion while the forearm is passively pronated. Electrophisiologic tests reveal reduced conductions and are generally not necessary for diagnosis.

8.5.3. Treatment

Surgical decompression using a dorsoradial approach. The superficial radial nerve is identified and released at it emerges beneath the brachioradialis tendon. The prognosis is excellent.

9. Conclusion

Compression neuropathies are one of the most prevalent disorders of the peripheral nervous system with an increasing incidence over the past decades. Recent studies have helped clarify the diagnosis and treatment for many of these neuropathies, facilitating a prompt recognition of the signs and symptoms, achieving an accurate diagnosis and a prompt treatment before the establishment of complications. The ability to recognize nerve entrapment syndromes and to distinguish them from other diseases of peripheral nerves, are important clinical skills. Although electrophysiological assessments are important in the diagnosis of neuropathies, our clinical skills remain the most reliable tool to identifying them and start an accurate treatment protocol. It is always important to begin with a non-operative strategy in patients with mild symptoms, nevertheless, surgical decompression is the definitive treatment of choice for most of the compression neuropathies, that is why it is important to know all the surgical alternatives and know the surgical anatomy for each upper extremity nerve.

Author details

Javier López Mendoza and Alexandro Aguilera Salgado

Postgraduate Course in Plastic and Reconstructive Surgery, Universidad Nacional Autónoma de México, Hospital General "Dr. Manuel Gea González", México City, Mexico

References

[1] David Warwick, MD. Compression Neuropathy. In: Oxford University Press. Oxford Specialist Handbooks in Surgery. Hand Surgery. (2009). , 314-331.

http://dx.doi.org/10.5772/55316

[2] Charles, H, & Thorne, M. D. Compression Neuropathies in the Upper Limb and Electrophisiologic Studies. In: Lippincott Williams & Wilkins. Grabb and Smith's Plastic Surgery. Sixth Edition. (2007). , 849-853.

[3] Robert, J, & Spinner, M. D. Compressive neuropathies of the upper extremity. Clin Plastic Surg (2003). , 30(2003), 155-173.

[4] David Green MD. Compression Neuropathies. In: Churchill Livingstone. El Sevier. Green's Operative Hand Surgery. (2005). Fifth Edition. , 999-1045.

[5] Karol, A, & Gutowski, M. D. Hand II: Peripheral Nerves and Tendon Transfers. In: Selected Readings in Plastic Surgery. (2003). , 9(33), 19-32.

[6] Brian McNamara, MD. Clinical Anatomy Of The Median Nerve. ACNR (2003). http://www.acnr.co.uk/pdfs/volume2pdfaccessed 19 August 2012).

[7] Akira NaganoSpontaneous Anterior Interroseous Nerve Palsy. The Journal Of Bone And Joint Surgery. (2003). B:313-8., 85.

[8] Spinner, M. Injuries to the Major Branches of Peripheral Nerves of the Forearm. Philadelphia: Saunders, (1978). , 160-227.

[9] Douglas, H. C. L. Anterior Interosseous Nerve Syndrome. Journal of The American Society For Surgery of the Hand. November (2001). , 1(4)

[10] American Academy of Orthopaedic Surgeons Work Group PanelClinical guidelines on diagnosis of carpal tunnel syndrome. Available at: www.aaos.org/research/guidelines/CTS_guideline.pdf.Accessed November 27, (2012).

[11] Jaimie, T, & Shores, M. D. An Evidence-Based Approach to Carpal Tunnel Syndrome. Plast. Reconstr. Surg. (2010). , 126, 2196-2204.

[12] Massy-westropp, N, Grimmer, K, & Bain, G. A systematic review of the clinical diagnostic tests for carpal tunnel syndrome. J Hand Surg (2000). A:, 120-127.

[13] Kyle, D, & Bickel, M. D. Carpal Tunnel Syndrome. J Hand Surg (2010). A:, 147-152.

[14] Robinson, L. R. Electrodiagnosis of Carpal Tunnel Syndrome. Phys Med Rehabil Clin N Am. Nov (2007).

[15] Zagnoli, F, & Andre, V. Le Dreff P, et al. Idiopathic Carpal Tunnel Syndrome. Clinical, electrodiagnostic, and magnetic resonance imaging correlations. Rev Rhum Engl Ed. Apr (1999). , 66(4), 192-200.

[16] Lee, D, Van Holsbeeck, M. T, Janevski, P. K, et al. Diagnosis of Carpal Tunnel Syndrome. Ultrasound Versus Electromyography. Radiol Clin North Am. Jul (1999). , 37(4), 859-72.

[17] Scholten, R. J. Mink van der Molen A, Uitdehaag BM, Bouter LM, de Vet HC. Surgical treatment options for carpal tunnel syndrome. Cochrane Database Syst Rev (2007). CD003905.

[18] Trumble, T. E, Diao, E, Abrams, R. A, & Gilbert-anderson, M. M. Single-portal endoscopic carpal tunnel release compared with open release: A prospective, randomized trial. J Bone Joint Surg Am. (2002). A:1107-1115., 84.

[19] Atroshi, I, Larsson, G. U, Ornstein, E, Hofer, M, Johnsson, R, & Ranstam, J. Outcomes of endoscopic surgery compared with open surgery for carpal tunnel syndrome among employed patients: Randomised controlled trial. BMJ. (2006).

[20] Mackinnon, S. E, Mccabe, S, Murray, J. F, et al. Internal neurolysis fails to improve the results of primary carpal tunnel decompression. J Hand Surg Am 16:211-218, (1991).

[21] Charlotte Shum, MD et al. The Role of Flexor Tenosynovectomy in the Operative Treatment of Carpal Tunnel Syndrome. The Journal of Bone and Joint Surgery (American) 84:221-225 ((2002).

[22] Daniel, B, & Polatsch, M. D. Ulnar Nerve Anatomy. Hand Clin (2007). , 23(2007), 283-289.

[23] Gonzalez, M. H, Lotfi, P, Bendre, A, & Mandelbroyt, Y. Lieska N: The ulnar nerve at the elbow and its local branching: An anatomic study. J Hand Surg [Br] 26B:(2001). , 142-144.

[24] Jason, H, & Huang, M. D. Ulnar Nerve Entrapment Neuropathy At The Elbow: Simple Decompression. Neurosurgery. (2004). , 55, 1150-1153.

[25] Lowe JB III, Maggi SP, Mackinnon SE. The position of crossing branches of the medial antebrachial cutaneous nerve during cubital tunnel surgery in humans. Plast Reconstr Surg (2004). , 114(3), 692-6.

[26] Keith, L. Moore. Arm, Forearm and Hand. In: Lippincott Williams & Wilkins. Anatomy With Clinical Orientation. (2004). Fourth Edition. , 730-796.

[27] Brian Rinker, MD. Proximal Radial Compression Neuropathy. Ann Plast Surg (2004). , 52, 174-180.

[28] Lister, G. D, Belsole, R. B, & Kleinert, H. E. The radial tunnel syndrome. J Hand Surg. (1979). , 4, 52-59.

Chapter 5

Postural Balance and Peripheral Neuropathy

Kathrine Jáuregui-Renaud

Additional information is available at the end of the chapter

http://dx.doi.org/10.5772/55344

1. Introduction

1.1. Control of posture

Postural control can be defined as the control of the body's position in space for the purposes of balance and orientation [1]. A definition of balance is the ability to maintain or return the body's centre of gravity within the limits of stability that are determined by the base of support (i.e., the area of the feet) [2]; while spatial orientation defines our natural ability to maintain our body orientation in relation to the surrounding environment, in static and dynamic conditions.

Maintaining balance encompasses the acts of preserving, achieving or restoring the body centre of mass relative to the limits of stability that are given by the base of support [3], which implies the control of posture in preventing falling. Then, in order to modify motor responses on the basis of sensory input, the appropriate responses to any external or internal perturbation have to be chosen [4]. Nevertheless, to maintain stability, all movements that affect the static and dynamic position of the center of mass of the body must be preceded or accompanied by adjustments of other segments.

During upright stance, balance corrections appear to be triggered by signals presumably located within the lower trunk or pelvis [5], and sensory feedback is required from vestibular, visual and somatosensory origin. A bipedal stance position that provides good stability is maintained mainly by efferent ankle mechanisms; to minimize the effect of perturbations when segmental oscillation is allowed, hip mechanisms are used. Locations of the centre of gravity at the borders of the limits of stability correspond to the region where balance cannot be maintained without moving the feet [6].

In order to orient the body, while keeping balance, visual, vestibular and somatosensory modalities are also involved. Every directed activity implies that the body was previously oriented [7]. Although, any part of the body surface can influence the control and perception of body orientation [8], evidence suggest that the representation of the body's static and dynamic geometry may be largely based on muscle proprioceptive inputs that continuously inform the central nervous system about the position of each part of the body in relation to the others [9-11]. The muscle innervation patterns necessary to produce particular body relative movements depend on body orientation to gravity [12]. To oppose the acceleration of gravity, there are contact forces of support on the body surface, the otolith organs provide information about head orientation with respect to the gravitoinertial force. If the head or both the head and the trunk are aligned with the vertical, the gravitational or egocentric reference associated with vertical gravity provide a strong spatial invariant used to control balance [13].

The attentional demands of postural control vary according to the postural task [14], the age of individuals and their balance abilities [15-17]. Teasdale et al. (1993) [18], examined the extent to which reduction in available sensory inputs may increase the attentional demands of postural control in healthy aduls; both young and old adults showed delays in reaction time as the postural task complexity increased, with an increase on attentional demands when sensory inputs were reduced. Studies using dual task paradigms to examine attention requirements of balance control when performing a secondary task, in both healthy and older adults with balance impairment, suggest that these are important contributions to instability, depending on the complexity of the task as well as the type of the second task being performed [15,17].

2. Afferent contributions to control posture

The maintenance of bipedal stance is characterized by continuous, small deviations around the actual upright. Depending on sensory context and neuromuscular constraints, the nervous system can adjust the relative afferent contributions to maintain stability. Evidence supports that, as we move about a changing environment, the nervous system continually integrates multisensory information, with the need for continual online updating of estimates of the centre of mass [19].

Balance corrections imply the interaction among several sensory inputs. Somatosensory systems respond early to motion and muscle stretch at the ankle, knee and trunk, as does the vestibular system, which senses head accelerations [20]. Visual inputs mainly influence later stabilizing reactions to the initial balance corrections [20-21]. Each sensory modality makes a unique contribution to control posture. However, the information sent by discrete receptors is not as relevant as the integrated information sent by receptors distributed throughout the body. Descending postural commands are multivariate in nature, and the motion at each joint is affected uniquely by input from multiple sensors. In different sensory environments, the nervous system is able to re-weight its available afferents in order to optimize stance control. For example, with increasing stance width, lateral body motion is detected more easily by proprioceptors and less readily by vision or the vestibular system [22].

http://dx.doi.org/10.5772/55344

Allum et al. have suggested that a confluence of knee, trunk and vestibulo-spinal inputs triggers human balance corrections depending on the mode of movement the body is forced into by a perturbation, and on the differential weighting of proprioceptive and vestibulo-spinal inputs in the triggered muscle's balance correcting response [5]. A combined deficit of vestibular and somatosensory input may preclude adjustments to postural control [23].

Normal postural coordination of the trunk and legs also requires both somatosensory and visual information [24]; older adults may be less stable under conditions in which peripheral vision is occluded and ankle somatosensation is limited, only remaining foveal vision and vestibular input [25]. However, evidence suggest different selection of sensory orientation references depending on the personal experience of the subjects, leading to a more or less heavy dependence on vision [26].

2.1. Somatosensory systems

When healthy subjects stand on a solid base of support, in a lightened environment, they rely on their somatosensory systems, the proprioceptive and the tactile systems. For this purpose, the proprioceptive system provides information on joint angles, changes in joint angles, joint position and muscle length and tension; while the tactile system is associated mainly with sensations of touch, pressure and vibration. In children, studies on the development of sensory organization to control posture according to each sensory component in relation to age suggests that the proprioceptive function seems to mature at 3 to 4 years of age [27].

During upright stance, somatosensory information from the legs may be utilized for both, direct sensory feedback and use of prior experience in scaling the magnitude of automatic postural responses [28]. Reduced somatosensory information from the lower limbs alters the ability to trigger postural responses and to scale the magnitude of these responses [29-31]. Even if the input from skin, pressure and joint receptors of the foot may be of minor importance for the compensation of rapid displacements, it may play a major role at low frequencies [32].

In patients with diabetic neuropathy, sensory conduction in the lower legs results in the late onset of an otherwise intact, centrally programmed response; along with this finding, a different relationship between the severity of the neuropathy and the quality of amplitude and velocity scaling suggests that the role of this peripheral sensory information may differ depending both, on the postural control task and on the quality of the sensory information available [28].

The foot sole and ankle muscle inputs contribute jointly to posture regulation [33]. Foot sole sensation is an important component of the balance system [34]. Cutaneous afferent messages from the main supporting zones of the feet may have sufficient spatial relevance to induce adapted regulative postural responses [35]. After perceptual training for hardness discrimination of the support surface, the ability of healthy subjects to regulate their standing posture may improve with improvement of the perceptive ability of the soles [36].

In healthy subjects, increased severity of experimentally induced loss of plantar cutaneous sensitivity may be associated with greater postural sway; such an association could be affected by the availability of visual input and the size of the support surface [37]. Additionally, subthreshold mechanical noise may enhance the detection of pressure changes on the sole of the feet [38].

Clinical studies have shown that patients with large-fibre neuropathy do not show abnormal body sway during stance [39-40]. Studies in patients with Charcot-Marie-Tooth type 1A disease suggest that functional integrity of the largest afferent fibres may not be necessary for appropriate equilibrium control during quiet stance [39]; also, in this group of patients, postural instability correlates significantly with decreased vibration [41].

Contact of the index finger with a stationary surface can greatly attenuate postural instability during upright stance, even when the level of force applied is far below that necessary to provide mechanical support [42]. In healthy subjects, standing in the dark, spatial information about body posture derived from fingertip contact with a stationary surface greatly improves stability [42]. However, haptic information about postural sway derived from contact with other parts of the body can also increase stability [43].

2.2. Visual system

Visual influence on postural control results from a complex synergy that receives multimodal inputs, and may have similar effects on the leg and trunk segments [44]. In order to stabilize the head in space, visual information of the environment must be definite [45]. Healthy subjects show decreased stability in the dark [46], and to compensate for large postural instabilities, visual information is required.

In infants, a cephalo-caudal developmental gradient may be observed as children develope from 3 to 14 months of age, while a wide variety of response patterns may be seen in the 3- to 5-month-olds, indicating that postural responses are not functional prior to experience with stabilizing the center of mass [47]. In children, the peripheral visual contribution to dynamic balance control increase from 3 to 6 years of age, with a maximum in 6-year-old children.; then it decreases in the 7-year-old children and increase again from 8–9 years of age to adulthood [48]. Evidence on the development of sensory organization to control posture, according to each sensory component, in relation to age suggests that the visual afferent system reach adult level at 15 to 16 years of age [27].

Epidemiological studies have shown that visual impairment is strongly associated with falls in the elderly [49-50]. Among older adults with glaucoma, greater visual field loss or thinner retinal nerve fiber layer thickness is associated with reduced postural stability [51]. These findings could be explained by several factors, including poor visual acuity, reduced visual field, impaired contrast sensitivity, and the presence of cataract [49, 52]. However, the role of vision in posture control may be evident even in subjects between 40 and 60 years old [53].

Visual inputs distinguish between translation and rotation of the head. Static visual cues may slowly control re-orientation or displacement, whereas dynamic visual cues may contribute to fast stabilization of the body [54]. Optical motions, like those produced when an observer moves through an environment, have an effect on postural stability [55}. However, flow structure apparently interacts with the exposed retinal area in controlling stance [56].

2.3. Vestibular system

Vestibular inputs tonically activate the anti-gravity leg muscles during normal standing

During dynamic tasks, vestibular information contributes to head stabilization to enable successful gaze control [57] and, during active tasks, it provides a stable reference frame from which to generate postural responses [13]. In children, evidence on the development of sensory organization to control posture, according to each sensory component in relation to age suggests that the vestibular afferent system reach adult level at 15 to 16 years of age [27].

Since loss of vestibular information may lead to deficits in trunk control but had less effect on the legs, vestibulo-spinal control may act primarily to stabilize the trunk in space and to facilitate intersegmental dynamics [58]. Vestibular influences are earlier for the sagittal plane and are directed to leg muscles, whereas roll control, in the frontal plane, is later and focused on trunk muscles [59]. Vestibular reflexes and perceptual signals appear to have a specific role in the maintenance of upright stance, under conditions in which other sources of postural information are attenuated or absent [60].

Patients with chronic unilateral peripheral loss may vary widely in the amount they could use their remaining vestibular function and show an increased reliance on proprioceptive information [61]. In patients with bilateral loss of vestibular function, postural compensation depends upon the ability to increase reliance on the remaining sensory systems for postural orientation [62]. During visually induced sway, patients with loss of vestibular function may not utilize somatosensory cues to a greater extent than normal subjects; that is, changes in somatosensory system gain may not be used to compensate for their vestibular deficit [63}. However, precision contact of the index finger at mechanically non-supportive force levels may serve as a substitute in subjects with vestibular loss, when they are attempting to maintain quiet stance [64].

3. Motor contribution to control posture

According to the review by Massion (1984) [65], posture is built up by the sum of several basic mechanisms. First the tone of the muscles gives them a rigidity that helps to maintain the joints in a defined position; the postural tone is added to this basic tonus, mainly in the extensor muscles. Postural fixation maintains the position of one or several joints against an internal force (eg. body weight), by co-contraction of the antagonistic muscles around the joints. Coordination between movement and posture is observed with the voluntary movements of body segments. Postural adjustments accompanying voluntary movements show three main characteristics [65]: they are anticipatory with respect to movement, they are adaptable to the condition in which the movement is executed and they are influenced by instructions given to the subjects concerning the task to be performed

During upright stance, compensatory torques must be generated to oppose the destabilizing torque due to gravity. Then, spontaneous sway is generated by the continuous body deviations countered by corrective torques. During movement of one segment of the body, other segments are disturbed, producing instability. Thus the precise movement of distal segments can be realized only by stabilizing more proximal segments [66]. Just before a voluntary movement, the stretch reflex response in agonist muscles is enhanced [67], consistent with a stabilizing effect. In healthy subjects, axial tone is modulated sensitively and dynamically, this control originates, at least in part, from tonic lengthening and shortening reactions, and a similar type of control appears to exist for postural tone in the proximal muscles of the arm [68].

To preserve balance, postural adjustments are made through flexible synergies, in which the activity of the participating muscles is set to task-specific conditions [5]. The most rapid postural reactions are a class of motor activities mediated primarily by inputs derived from the forces and motions of the feet upon the surface of support [69]; the supporting reactions and placing reactions (tactile, visual and vestibular) adapt the activity of the postural muscles of the limbs to their function of body support. Perturbations to balance imply that the central nervous system select patterns of muscle activation that are appropriate for a variety of perturbations [70], in agreement with biomechanical constraints such as those imposed by inter-segmental dynamics and musculoskeletal geometry [71]. A confluence of proprioceptive and vestibular modulation to the basic centrally initiated template of activity may establish the amplitude pattern of the muscle response synergy [70, 72-73]. The confluence of sensory inputs presumably permits the proprioceptive and vestibular inputs to reinforce each other righting effects, and prevent to fall.

It has been suggested that postural adjustments can be described as a single feedback control scheme, with scalable heterogenic gains that are adjusted according to biomechanical constraints [74]. In addition, muscle weakness and muscle fatigue have to be considered. Clinical evidence have shown that patients with polyneuropathy who have ankle weakness are more likely to experience multiple and injurious falls than are those without specific muscle weakness [75]. Also, an altered posture, which is common in patients with muscle weakness, may interfere with the position of the centre of mass, and there by also cause balance problems [76].

In healthy subjects, inducing localized muscle fatigue at various musculatures has been shown to adversely affect postural control. Plantar-flexor muscle fatigue may impair the effectiveness of postural control and increase the amount of postural regulatory activity required to control unperturbed bipedal posture when the quality of the postural support surface information is altered (by standing on a foam support surface) to a greater extent than when it is not [77]. In healthy subjects who perform fatiguing exercises, acute effects of fatigue may differ between joints, with the most substantial effects evident at the lower back, followed by the ankle and recovery of postural control [78]. Also, during quiet standing, fatigue of trunk muscles may increase reliance on somatosensory inputs from the foot soles and ankles for controlling posture [79], while lumbar fatigue impairs the ability to sense a change in lumbar position [80].

4. Clinical assessment of balance

In order to assess instability or walking difficulty, it is essential to identify the affected movements and circumstances in which they occur (i.e. uneven surfaces, environmental light, activity) as well as any other associated clinical manifestation that could be related to balance, postural control, motor control, muscular force, movement limitations or sensory deficiency.

The clinical evaluation should include a detailed assessment of long tracts, cranial nerves, motor control, motor strength, the eyes and the ears. To evaluate the vestibular system and its relationships with other sensory inputs and the oculo-motor system, specific tests have to be performed, including eye movement recordings and vestibular reflexes.

Standardized scales and questionnaires may be helpful to evaluate and to follow-up deficits that may be evident on daily life activities (e.i. Berg's Balance Scale [81]; Tinetti scale [82]; balance symptoms questionnaire by Jáuregui-Renaud et al.[83]), as well as falls [84]. Some clinical test include the "Get up and go test" [85], the five-step test and the Functional Reach [86], the Mobility Fall Chart [87] and the evidence based risk assessment tool [88], among others. However, before choosing a tool the clinician should consider the purpose of its design and the purpose for which the tool is to be applied, as well as its reliability.

To evaluate balance, a neurological examination should be performed, including an examination of motor and sensory function; care should be taken to assess static and dynamic postural control and gait, as well as to identify visual and vestibular disorders. During static upright stance, it is important to observe the width of the stance, the symmetry of the stance, the balance at the level of the joints as well as the trunk posture, while changing the sensory conditions (i.e. visual input and the surface of support). The sensory conditions may include at least: standing with the eyes open and closed, on a hard and a compliant surface, standing with the feet together and balancing on the two legs. To clinically asses the response to simple perturbations, the clinician may observe the reaction to push gently the patient while standing.

To measure balance, different aspects may be analysed: electric potentials due to muscle activation, kinematics that is concerned with movement itself and kinetics, concerned with the forces and the moments of forces that are developed during movements. To record kinetics, force platforms are used. The centre of pressure is recorded over a period of time, while standing on the force platform (wearing a safety harness) under different sensory conditions. Several moving force platforms have been designed in order to create dynamic conditions, while maintaining a constant angle between the foot and lower leg and moving the visual enclosure of the platform, which can be coupled to the body sway. Regardless of the technique of measurement used, to interpret any recording of body sway, several factors have to be considered, including the fact that body sway increase with age, with an increased dependence on vision [53, 89-90], and may be affected by body weight and gender [90-91]. In patients with polyneuropathy, special care should be taken in considering adaptive compensation to changes in biomechanical factors as well as sensory deficits.

To evaluate gait, a sensory-motor evaluation should be performed, as well as a postural and skeletal examination [92]. To asses walking it is necessary to analyse the initiation, the stepping, the termination and the associated movements. During stepping, it is important to evaluate at least the speed of walking, the rhythm and the length of each stride.

The analysis of gait may include measurements of joint kinematics and kinetics, other measurements include electromyography, oxygen consumption and foot pressures. Using electromyography, specific muscles or muscle groups during movement can be studied. A kinematic evaluation (e.i. joint angles, stride length, walking velocity) may be performed by optoelectric methods as well as by tracking the position of the body segments using light-emitting markers. Power is a kinetic variable, to assess the rate of work performed at a given joint [93], which allows to identify when the muscle is generating or absorbing mechanical energy (concentric or eccentric contraction).

5. Balance in patients with peripheral neuropathy

Patients with polyneuropathy, which reduces sensation and often strength in the lower extremities, may have decreased stability while standing and when subjected to dynamic balance conditions [28, 94-97]. In patients with severe peripheral neuropathy of unknown origin, compared to healthy age and sex matched controls, visual and vestibular input cannot fully compensate for the impairment in proprioception, with progressive deterioration of balance [31].

The ability to re-weight sensory information depending on the sensory context is important for maintaining stability, when an individual moves from one sensory context to another, such as a flat walking surface to an uneven surface or a well-lit sidewalk to a dimly lit garden. Individuals with peripheral vestibular loss or somatosensory loss from neuropathy are limited in their ability to re-weight postural sensory dependence [31, 98].

In patients with peripheral neuropathy, including Charcot-Marie-Tooth disease type 1A and type 2 and diabetic neuropathy, the effects of impaired proprioceptive input in balance control under static and dynamic conditions [99] showed that, during static conditions, across all patients, instability increased as a function of the slowing of conduction velocity. In contrast, during dynamic conditions head displacement was only slightly increased, compared to healthy subjects, despite the increased delay at which the head followed displacement of the feet.

Charcot–Marie–Tooth disease is a genetically heterogeneous group of hereditary neuropathies characterized by slowly progressive weakness and atrophy, primarily in the distal leg muscles. The clinical disability has been shown to best correlate with the degree of axonal loss [100]. However, evidence suggest that functional integrity of the largest afferent fibres is not necessary for appropriate equilibrium control during quiet stance, and unsteadiness is related to additional functional alterations in smaller fibres, most likely group II spindle afferent fibres [39].

In adult patients with Charcot–Marie-Tooth type 1A, the decline in axonal function and in muscle strength may reflect, to a considerable extent, a process of normal ageing, and

http://dx.doi.org/10.5772/55344

physical disability in adulthood may well be explained by decreased reserves and compensatory mechanisms together with progression of skeletal deformations due to muscle weakness [101]. On the other hand, during static conditions, patients with Charcot-Marie-Tooth type 2 may show less postural stability than patients with Charcot-Marie-Tooth type 1A disease, but similar than the postural stability shown by diabetic patients with peripheral neuropathy [99]; while in patients with diabetic peripheral neuropathy, unsteadiness relates to alterations in medium-size myelinated afferent fibres, possibly originating from spindle secondary terminations [40].

A frequent source of polyneuropathy is diabetes mellitus. Diabetic peripheral neuropathy is initially characterized by a reduction in somesthesic sensitivity due to the sensitive nerve damage, and with progression motor nerves are damaged. During upright stance, compared to healthy subjects, recordings of the centre of pressure in patients with diabetic neuropathty have shown larger sway [95-96, 102], as well as increased oscillation at 0.5-1 Hz [103]. However, in this group of patients, in addition to postural instability caused by neuropathy, balance deterioration may also result from the bio-mechanical impairment caused by progression of foot complications [104], as well as from the compromise of other sensory inputs such as vision [105-106]. Compared to healthy subjects, diabetic patients may have poorer balance during standing in diminished light compared to full light and no light conditions [105].

Balance and gait difficulties are the most frequently cited cause of falling in all age and gender groups [107] A fall is often defined as inadvertently coming to rest on the ground, floor or other lower level, excluding intentional change in position to rest in furniture, wall or other objects [108]. Cavanagh et al. (1992) [109] have shown that, compared to patients with diabetes but no peripheral neuropathy, patients with diabetic peripheral neuropathy are more likely to report an injury during walking or standing, which may be more frequent when walking on irregular surfaces [110].

Epidemiological surveys have established that a reduction of leg proprioception is a risk factor for falls in the elderly [111-112]. Symptoms and signs of peripheral neuropathy are frequently found during physical examination of older subjects. These clinical manifestations may be related to diabetes mellitus, alcoholism, nutritional deficiencies, autoimmune diseases, among other causes. In this group of patients, loss of plantar sensation may be an important contributor to the dynamic balance deficits and increased risk of falls [34, 109].

Falls occur as a result of complex interactions among demographic, physical and behavioural factors. Risk factors may be intrinsic or extrinsic: intrinsic factors include demographic and biological factors, while extrinsic factors encompass environmental and behavioural factors [108]. Among other risk factors, the occurrence of falls may be significantly associated with lower extremity weakness, which can be measured by knee extension, ankle dorsiflexion, and chair stands [113], visual acuity of less than 6/12 [114], lower extremity impairments [108-109] and poly-pharmacy [115-116].

Apart from sensorymotor compromise, fear of falling may relate to restriction and avoidance of activities, which results in loss of strength especially in the lower extremities, and may also be predictive for future falls [117-119].

6. Interventions to improve balance in patients with peripheral neuropathy

Richardson et al. (2004) [120], in patients with various forms of peripheral neuropathy, found that the use of a cane, ankle orthoses or touching a wall improved spatial and temporal measures of gait regularity while walking under challenging conditions. Evidence support that, additional hand contact of external objects may reduce postural instability caused by a deficiency of one or more senses. Contact with support of varying stability may reduce the destabilizing effect of a moving visual scene [121]. In patients with moderate to severe diabetic neuropathy, mechanical noise stimulation may improve vibration and tactile perception [122].

To improve stability in patients with decreased somatosensation, footwear may represent a modifiable factor. The efficacy of certain types of stabilizing reactions may be improved whether incorporating a pressure plantar-based biofeedback system in footwear [123], vibrating shoe insoles [38], or by mechanical facilitation of sensation from the boundaries of the plantar surface of the foot [124]. In patients with Charcot-Marie-Tooth, considering individual sensory and muscular deficits, ankle-foot orthosis prescription, appears relevant for improving balance and gait performance [125].

Exercise that improves lower-extremity balance and strength (force-generating capacity) has been shown to be effective in reducing falls in older adults [126]. In patients with clinically defined sensory ataxia due to bilateral chronic neuropathy compared to patients with unilateral loss-related to multiple sclerosis, after a rehabilitation program including foot sensory stimulation, balance and gait training with limited vision, balance assessed on a static force platform remained similar in the open-eyes condition and improved in the closed-eyes condition only in patients with unilateral sensory loss, while dynamic balance improved in the two groups, suggesting that the relative contribution of proprioceptive and visual inputs may depend on the extent of somatosensory loss [127].

Guidelines for diabetes management recommend that patients perform at least 30 min of physical activity a day six times a week. Few studies on prevention of diabetic neuropathy through exercise have been reported, even if moderate intensity exercise in patients with type 2 diabetes mellitus has been associated with a decrease in blood glucose [128]. A preliminary controlled study has shown that a 12 week program of *tai chi chuan* exercises may improve peripheral nerve conduction velocities and fasting glucose levels [129].

Studies evaluating treatment strategies that could improve balance in diabetic patients with polyneuropathy are also scarce. Although, some interventions including leg strengthening and balance exercises to promote ambulatory physical activity may not decrease fall rates, but neither they increase them; suggesting that physical activity interventions that increase activity probably do not increase the risk of falling in patients with diabetic peripheral neuropathy [130]. In this group of patients, specific training may improve gait speed, balance, muscle strength and joint mobility [131].

To determine the effect of a specific exercise regimen on clinical measures of postural stability and confidence in a population with peripheral neuropathy, compared to a control group, ten patients with diabetic peripheral neuropathy underwent a 3-week intervention to increase rapidly available distal strength and balance, showing improvement on unipedal stance time, functional reach, tandem stance time, but the score on the activities-specific balance and confidence scale [132]. To further increase physical activity and protocol adherence, a supervised centre-based exercise program rather than a self-administered program may be recommended [130]. However, there is a need of studies examining the effect of physical training on the incidence of foot breakdown and fall risk in people with diabetes mellitus and peripheral neuropathy.

7. Conclusions

Postural control can be defined as the control of the body’s position in space for the purposes of balance and orientation. Balance is the ability to maintain or return the body's centre of gravity within the limits of stability that are determined by the base of support. Spatial orientation defines our natural ability to maintain our body orientation in relation to the surrounding environment, in static and dynamic conditions.

The representation of the body's static and dynamic geometry may be largely based on muscle proprioceptive inputs that continuously inform the central nervous system about the position of each part of the body in relation to the others. Posture is built up by the sum of several basic mechanisms. First the tone of the muscles gives them a rigidity that helps to maintain the joints in a defined position; the postural tone is added to this basic tonus. Postural fixation maintains the position of one or several joints against an internal force. During movement of one segment of the body, other segments are disturbed, producing instability. Thus the precise movement of distal segments can be realized only by stabilizing more proximal segments.

Postural balance is dependent upon integration of signals from the somatosensory, visual and vestibular systems, to generate motor responses, with cognitive demands that vary according to the task, the age of the individuals and their ability to balance. Descending postural commands are multivariate in nature, and the motion at each joint is affected uniquely by input from multiple sensors.

The proprioceptive system provides information on joint angles, changes in joint angles, joint position and muscle length and tension; while the tactile system is associated mainly with sensations of touch, pressure and vibration.

Visual influence on postural control results from a complex synergy that receives multimodal inputs. Vestibular inputs tonically activate the anti-gravity leg muscles and, during dynamic tasks, vestibular information contributes to head stabilization to enable successful gaze control, providing a stable reference frame from which to generate postural responses.

In order to assess instability or walking difficulty, it is essential to identify the affected movements and circumstances in which they occur (i.e. uneven surfaces, environmental light, activity) as well as any other associated clinical manifestation that could be related to balance, postural control, motor control, muscular force, movement limitations or sensory deficiency. The clinical evaluation should include neurological examination; special care should be taken to identify visual and vestibular disorders, and to assess static and dynamic postural control and gait. Standardized scales and questionnaires may be helpful to evaluate and to follow-up deficits that may be evident on daily life activities.

The simplest method to record postural sway uses a force plate to measure the feet centre of pressure on the platform. To modify the somatosensory and visual inputs, moving force platforms and visual surroundings have been designed. Gait analysis may include the measurement of joint kinematics and kinetics, electromyography, oxygen consumption and foot pressures.

Polyneuropathy modify the amount and the quality of the sensorial information that is necessary for motor control, with increased instability during both, upright stance and gait.

Patients with peripheral neuropathy may have decreased stability while standing and when subjected to dynamic balance conditions. During upright stance, compared to healthy subjects, recordings of the centre of pressure in patients with diabetic neuropathy have shown larger sway, as well as increased oscillation at 0.5-1 Hz.

Balance and gait difficulties are the most frequently cited cause of falling in all age and gender groups Epidemiological surveys have established that a reduction of leg proprioception is a risk factor for falls.

Patients with polyneuropathy who have ankle weakness are more likely to experience multiple and injurious falls than are those without specific muscle weakness.

Elderly patients with diabetic peripheral neuropathy are more likely to report an injury during walking or standing, which may be more frequent when walking on irregular surfaces. Among other risk factors, the occurrence of falls may be significantly associated with lower extremity weakness, which can be measured by knee extension, ankle dorsiflexion, and chair stands, visual acuity of less than 6/12, lower extremity impairments and poly-pharmacy, among other factors.

In patients with various forms of peripheral neuropathy, the use of a cane, ankle orthoses or touching a wall improved spatial and temporal measures of gait regularity while walking under challenging conditions. Additional hand contact of external objects may reduce postural instability caused by a deficiency of one or more senses.

Studies evaluating preventive and treatment strategies through excercise that could improve balance in patients with polyneuropathy are scarce. However, evidence support that physical activity interventions that increase activity probably do not increase the risk of falling in patients with diabetic peripheral neuropathy, and in this group of patients, specific training may improve gait speed, balance, muscle strength and joint mobility.

http://dx.doi.org/10.5772/55344

Author details

Kathrine Jáuregui-Renaud

Instituto Mexicano del Seguro Social, México

References

[1] Shumway-Cook A, Woollacott M. Motor Control: Theory and Practical Applications (2nd edition).Baltimore: Lippincott, Williams and Wilkins; 2000.

[2] Horak FB. Clinical measurement of postural control in adults. Physical Therapy 1987; 67(12):1881-1885.

[3] Pollock A, Durward BR, Rowe PJ, Paul JP. What is balance? Clinical Rehabilitation 2000;14(4):402-406.

[4] Era P, Schroll M, Ytting H, Gause-Nilsson I, Heikkinen E, Steen B. Postural balance and its sensory motor correlates in 75-year-old men and women: A cross-national comparative study. Journals of Gerontology. Series A, Biological Sciences and Medical Sciences 1996; 51(2):M53 -M63.

[5] Allum JH, Bloem BR, Carpenter MG, Hulliger M, Hadders-Algra M. Proprioceptive control of posture: a review of new concepts. Gait & Posture 1998; (3):214–242.

[6] Horak FB, Shupert CL, Mirka A. Components of postural sway dyscontrol in the elderly: a review. Neurobiology of Aging 1989;10(6):727-738.

[7] Gurfinkel VS, Levick YS. Perceptual and automatic aspects of the postural body scheme. In: Paillard J (ed). Brain and space. New York: Oxford University Press; 1991.

[8] Lackner JR. Some contributions of touch, pressure and kinesthesis to human spatial orientation and oculomotor control. Acta Astronautautica 1981; 8 (8):825-830.

[9] Massion J. Movement, posture and equilibrium: interaction and coordination. Progress in Neurobiology 1992;38:35-56.

[10] Roll JP, Vedel JP, Roll R. Eye, head and squeletal muscle spindle feedback in the elaboration of body references. Progress in Brain Research 1989;80:113-123.

[11] Kavounoudias A, Gilhodes JC, Roll R, Roll J. From balance regulation to body orientation: two goals for muscle proprioceptive information processing? Experimental Brain Research 1999;124(1): 80-88.

[12] Lackner JR, Di Zio P. Human orientation and movement control in weightless and artificial gravity environments. Experimental Brain Research 2000;130(1):2–26.

[13] Pozzo T, Levik Y, Berthoz A. Head and trunk movements in the frontal plane during complex dynamic equilibrium tasks in humans. Experimental Brain Research 1995; 106(2): 327-338.

[14] Teasdale N, Simoneau M. Attentional demands for postural control: the effects of ageing and sensory reintegration. Gait & Posture 2001;14(3):203-210.

[15] Camicioli R, Howieson D, Lehman S. Talking while walking: the effect of a dual task in ageing and Alzheimer's disease. Neurology 1997;48(4):955-958.

[16] Kerr B, Condon SM, McDonald LA. Cognitive spatial processing and the regulation of posture. Journal of Experimental Psychology. Human Perception and Performance 1985;11 (5):617-622.

[17] Woollacott M, Shumway-Cook A. Attention and the control of posture and gait: a review of an emerging area of research. Gait & Posture 2002;16 (1):1-14.

[18] Teasdale N, Bard C, LaRue J, Fleury M. On the cognitive penetrability of postural control. Experimental Aging Research 1993;19(1):1–13.

[19] Oie KS, Kiemel T, Jeka JJ. Human multisensory fusion of vision and touch: detecting nonlinearity with small changes in the sensory environment. Neuroscience Letters 2001;315(3):113–116.

[20] Allum JH, Honegger F, Schicks H. Vestibular and proprioceptive modulation of postural synergies in normal subjects. Journal of Vestibular Research: Equilibrium & Orientation 1993; 3(1): 59-85.

[21] Allum JH, Pfaltz CR. Visual and vestibular contributions to pitch sway stabilization in the ankle muscles of normals and patients with bilateral vestibular deficits. Experimental Brain Research 1985;58(1):82–94.

[22] Day BL, Steiger MJ, Thompson PD, Marsden CD. Effect Of Vision And Stance Width On Human Body Motion When Standing: Implications For Afferent Control Of Lateral Sway. The Journal of Physiology1993;469):479-499.

[23] Aranda-Moreno C, Meza A, Rodriguez R, Mantilla MT, Jáuregui-Renaud K. Diabetic polyneuropathy may increase the handicap related to vestibular disease. Archives of Medical Research 2009;40(3):180-185.

[24] Kuo AD, Speers RA, Peterka RJ, Horak FB. Effect of altered sensory conditions on multivariate descriptors of human postural sway. Experimental Brain Research 1998; 122(2):185-195.

[25] Manchester D, Woollacott M, Zederbauer-Hylton N, Marin O. Visual, Vestibular and Somatosensory Contributions to Balance Control in the Older Adult. Journal of Gerontology 1989; 44(4):M118-M127.

[26] Lacour M, Barthelemy J, Borel L, Magnan J, Xerri C, Chays A, Ouaknine M. Sensory strategies in human postural control before and after unilateral vestibular neurotomy. Experimental Brain Research 1997;115(2):300-310.

[27] Steindl R, Kunz K, Schrott-Fischer A, Scholtz AW. Effect of age and sex on maturation of sensory systems and balance control. Developmental Medicine & Child Neurology 2006;48 (6):477-482.

[28] Inglis JT, Horak FB, Shupert ChL, Jones-Rycewicz C.The importance of somatosensory information in triggering and scaling automatic postural responses in humans. Experimental Brain Research 1994;101(1):159-164.

[29] Diener HC, Dichgans J, Bootz F, Bacher M. Early stabilization of human posture after a sudden disturbance: influence of rate and amplitude of displacement. Experimental Brain Research 1984b;56(1):126-134.

[30] Horak FB, Nashner LM, Diener .C. Postural strategies associated with somatosensory and vestibular loss. Experimental Brain Research 1990; 82(1):167-177.

[31] Jáuregui-Renaud K, Kovacsovics B, Vrethem M, Odjvist LM, Ledin T. Dynamic and Randomized perturbed posturography in the follow-up of patients with polyneuropathy. Archives of Medical Research 1998;29(1):39-44.

[32] Diener HC, Dichgans J, Guschlbauer B, Mau H. The significance of proprioception on postural stabilization as assessed by ischemia. Brain Research 1984a; 296(1): 103-109.

[33] Kavounoudias A, Roll R, Roll JP. Foot sole and ankle muscle inputs contribute jointly to human erect posture regulation. The Journal of Physiology 2001;5532 (3): 869-878.

[34] Meyer PF, Oddsson LI, De Luca CJ. Reduced plantar sensitivity alters postural responses to lateral perturbations of balance. Experimental Brain Research 2004; 157(4): 526-536.

[35] Kavounoudias A, Roll R, Roll JP. The plantar sole is a 'dynamometric map' for human balance control. Neuroreport 1998; 9(14):3247-3252.

[36] Morioka S, Yagi F. Influence of perceptual learning on standing posture balance: repeated training for hardness discrimination of foot sole. Gait & Posture 2004;20(1): 36-40.

[37] Wang TY, Lin I. Sensitivity of plantar cutaneous sensation and postural stability. Clinical Biomechanics (Bristol, Avon) 2008;23(4):493-499.

[38] Priplata A, Niemi J, Salen M, Harry J, Lipsitz LA, Collins JJ. Noise-enhanced human balance control. Physical Review Letters 2002; 89(23); 238101.

[39] Nardone A, Tarantola J, Miscio G, Pisano F, Schenone A, Schieppati M. Loss of large-diameter spindle afferent fibres is not detrimental to the control of body sway during upright stance: evidence from neuropathy. Experimental Brain Research 2000;135(2): 155-162.

[40] Nardone A, Schieppati M. Group II spindle fibres and afferent control of stance. Clues from diabetic neuropathy. Clinical Neurophysiology 2004;115(4):779-789.

[41] van der Linden MH, van der Linden SC, Hendricks HT, van Engelen BG, Geurts AC. Postural instability in Charcot-Marie-Tooth type 1A patients is strongly associated with reduced somatosensation. Gait & Posture 2010;31(4):483-488.

[42] Holden M, Ventura J, Lackner JR. Stabilization of posture by precision contact of the index finger. Journal of Vestibular Research: Equilibrium & Orientation 1994; 4(4): 285–301.

[43] Lackner JR, Rabin E, Di Zio P. Stabilization of posture by precision touch of the index finger with rigid and flexible filaments. Brain Research 2001;139 (4):454–464.

[44] Kiemel T, Zhang Y, Jeka JJ. Visual flow is interpreted relative to multisegment postural control. Journal of Motor Behavior 2011;43(3):237-246.

[45] Schmid M, Casabianca, L, Bottaro A, Schieppati M. Graded changes in balancing behavior as a function of visual acuity. Neuroscience 2008;153(4):1079-1091.

[46] Dichgans J, Brandt T. Visual-vestibular interaction, effects on self motion perception and postural control. In: Held R, Leibowitz H, Teuber HL (eds). Handbook of sensory physiology, Vol. VIII, perception. Berlin-New York: Springer Verlag. p 755–804.

[47] Woollacott M, Debu B, Mowatt M. Neuromuscular control of posture in the infant and child: is vision dominant? Journal of Motor Behavior 1987;19(2):167-186.

[48] Assaiante C, Amblard B. Peripheral vision and age-related differences in dynamic balance. Human Movement Science 1992;11(5):533–548.

[49] Ivers RQ, Cumming RG, Mitchell P, Attebo K. Visual impairment and falls in older adults: the Blue Mountains Eye Study. Journal of the American Geriatrics Society 1998;46(1):58-64.

[50] Tran TH, Nguyen Van Nuoi D, Baiz H, Baglin G, Leduc JJ, Bulkaen H. Visual impairment in elderly fallers. Journal français d'ophtalmologie, 2011;34(10):723-728.

[51] Black A, Wood JM, Lovie-Kitchin JE, Newman BM. Visual impairment and postural sway among older adults with glaucoma. Optometry and Visual Science 2008; 85(6): 489-497.

[52] Paulus WM, Straube A, Brandt T.Visual stabilization of posture. Physiological stimulus characteristics and clinical aspects. Brain 1984;107(Pt 4):1143-1163.

[53] Poulain I., Giraudet G. Age-related changes of visual contribution in posture control. Gait & Posture 2008; 27(1):1-7.

[54] Amblard B, Crémieux J, Marchand AR, Carblanc A. Lateral orientation and stabilization of human stance: static versus dynamic visual cues. Experimental Brain Research 1985;61(1): 21-37.

[55] Berthoz A, Pavard B, Young LR. Perception of linear horizontal self-motion induced by peripheral vision (linearvection). Experimental Brain Research 1975; 23(5):471-489.

[56] Stoffregen T. A.Flow structure versus retinal location in the optical control of stance. Journal of Experimental Psychology and Human Perception Performance 1985; 11(5): 554-565.

[57] Pozzo T, Berthoz A, Lefort L. Head stabilization during various locomotor tasks in humans: normal subjects. Experimental Brain Research 1990;82(1):97–106.

[58] Creath R, Kiemel T, Horak F, Jeka JJ. The role of vestibular and somatosensory systems in intersegmental control of upright stance. Journal of Vestibular Research: Equilibrium & Orientation 2008;18(1):39–49.

[59] Carpenter M, Allum J, Honegger F. Vestibular influences on human postural control in combinations of pitch and roll planes reveal differences in spatiotemporal processing. Experimental Brain Research 2001;140(1):95-111.

[60] Bacsi AM, Colebatch JG. Evidence for reflex and perceptual vestibular contributions to postural control. Experimental Brain Research 2005;160(1):22-28.

[61] Peterka RJ, Statler KD, Wrisley DM, Horak FB. Postural Compensation for Unilateral Vestibular Loss. Frontiers in Neurology 2011;2:57. doi:Â 10.3389/ fneur.2011.00057.

[62] Peterka RJ. Sensorimotor integration in human postural control. Journal of Neurophysiology 2002; 88(3):1097-1118.

[63] Peterka RJ, Benolken M. Role of somatosensory and vestibular cues in attenuating visually induced human postural sway. Experimental Brain Research 1995; 105(1): 101-110.

[64] Lackner, J.R., Di Zio, P., Jeka, J., Horak, F., Krebs, D., Rabin, E. Precision contact of the fingertip reduces postural sway of individuals with bilateral vestibular loss. Experimental Brain Research 1999;126(4):459–466.

[65] Massion J. Postural Changes Accompanying voluntary movements. Normal and pathological aspects. Human Neurobiology 1984;2(4):261-267.

[66] Hasan Z. The human motor control system's response to mechanical perturbation: should it, can it, and does it ensure stability? Journal of Motor Behavior 2005; 37(6): 484-493.

[67] Prochazka A. Sensorimotor gain control: A basic strategy of motor systems? Progress in Neurobiology 1989; 33:281-307.

[68] Gurfinkel V, Cacciatore TW, Cordo P, Horak F, Nutt J, Skoss R. Postural Muscle Tone in the Body Axis of Healthy Humans. Journal of Neurophysiology 2006;96(5): 2678-2687.

[69] Nashner LM. Fixed patterns of rapid postural responses among leg muscles during stance. Experimental Brain Research 1977; 30(1):13-24.

[70] Diener HC, Horak FB, Nashner LM. Influence of stimulus parameters on human postural responses. Journal of Neurophysiology 1988;59(6):1888-1905.

[71] Kuo, A.D., Zajac, F.E. A biomechanical analysis of muscle strength as a limiting factor in standing posture. Journal of Biomechanics 1993;26: 137–150.

[72] Forssberg H, Hirschfeld H. Postural adjustments in sitting humans following external perturbations: muscle activity and kinematics. Experimental Brain Research 1994; 97(3):515–527.

[73] Horak FB, Shupert CL, Dietz V, Horstmann G. Vestibular and somatosensory contributions to responses to head and body displacements in stance. Experimental Brain Research 1994;100(1):93-106.

[74] Park S, Horak F, Kuo A. Postural feedback responses scale with biomechanical constraints in human standing. Experimental Brain Research 2004;154(4) 417-427.

[75] Richardson JK. Factors associated with falls in older patients with diffuse polyneuropathy. Journal of the American Geriatrics Society 2002;50(11):1767-1773.

[76] Horlings CG, van Engelen BG, Allum JH, Bloem BR. A weak balance: the contribution of muscle weakness to postural instability and falls. Nat Clin Pract Neurol 2008;4(9):504-515.

[77] Hlavackovaa P, Vuillerme N. Do somatosensory conditions from the foot and ankle affect postural responses to plantar-flexor muscles fatigue during bipedal quiet stance? Gait & Posture 2012;36(1):16-19.

[78] Lin D, Nussbaum MA, Seol H, Singh NB, Madigan ML, Wojcik LA. Acute effects of localized muscle fatigue on postural control and patterns of recovery during upright stance: influence of fatigue location and age. European Journal of Applied Physiology 2009; 106(3):425-434.

[79] Vuillerme N, Chenu O, Pinsault N, Boisgontier, M., Demongeot, J., Payan, Y. Interindividual variability in sensory weighting of a plantar pressure-based, tongue-placed tactile biofeedback for controlling posture. Neuroscience Letters 2007:421 (2):173-177.

[80] Taimela S, Kankaanpää M, Luoto S. The effect of lumbar fatigue on the ability to sense a change in lumbar position. A controlled study. Spine (Phila Pa) 1976;25 (13): 1322-1327.

[81] Berg KO, Wood-Dauphinee SL, Williams JI, Maki BE. Measuring balance in the elderly: validation of an instrument. Canadian Journal of Public Health 1992;83 Suppl 2:S7-S11.

[82] Tinetti ME. Performance-oriented assessment of mobility problems in elderly patients. Journal of the American Geriatrics Society 1986;34 (2):119-126.

[83] Jáuregui-Renaud K, Gutierrez MA, Viveros RL, Villanueva PL. Síntomas de Inestabilidad Corporal y Enfermedad Vestibular. Revista Medica del Instituto Mexicano del Seguro Social 2003;41(5):373-378.

[84] Scott V, Votova K, Scanlan A, Close J. Multifactorial and functional mobility assessment tools for fall risk among older adults in community, home-support, long-term and acute care settings. Age and Ageing 2007:36(2)130–139.

[85] Podsiadlo D, Richardson S. The timed "Up & Go": a test of basic functional mobility for frail elderly persons. Journal of the American Geriatrics Society 1991;39(2): 142-148.

[86] Wang CY, Olson SL, Protas EJ. Physical-performance tests to evaluate mobility disability in community-dwelling elders. Journal of Aging and Physical Activity 2005;13(2)184-197.

[87] Lundin-Olsson L, Nyberg L, Gustafson Y. The mobility interaction fall chart. Physiotherapy Research International 2000;5(3):190–201.

[88] Oliver D, Britton M, Seed P, Martin FC, Hopper AH.Development and evaluation of evidence based risk assessment tool (STRATIFY) to predict which elderly inpatients will fall: case-control and cohort studies. BMJ 1997;315(7115):1049-1053.

[89] Colledge NR, Cantley P, Peaston I, Brash H, Lewis S, Wilson JA. Aging and balance: the measurement of spontanaeous sway by posturography. Gerontology 1994;40(5): 273-278.

[90] Era P, Sainio P, Koskinen S, Haavisto P, Vaara M, Aromaa A. Postural balance in a random sample of 7,979 subjects aged 30 years and over. Gerontology 2006: 52(4): 204-213.

[91] Cruz-Gómez NS, Plascencia G, Villanueva-Padrón LA, Jáuregui-Renaud K. Influence of obesity and gender on the postural stability during upright stance. Obesity Facts 2011;4(3):212-217.

[92] Thompson PD, Mardsen CD. Clinical Neurological assessment of balance and gait disorders. In: Bronstein A.M., Brandt T., Woollacott M. Clinical Disorders of Balance, Posture and Gait. London:Arnold;1996. p79-84.

[93] Mueller MJ, Minor SD, Sahrmann AS, Schaaf JA, Strube MJ. Differences in the gait characteristics of patients with diabetes and peripheral neuropathy compared with age-matched controls. Physical Therapy 1994;74 (4):299-313.

[94] Richardson JK, Ching C, Hurvitz EA. The relationship between electromyographically documented peripheral neuropathy and falls. Journal of the American Geriatrics Society 1992;40(10):1008-1112.

[95] Simoneau GG, Ulbrecht JS, Der JA, Becker MB, Cavanagh PR. Postural Instability in Patients with Diabetic Sensory Neuropathy. Diabetes Care 1994: 17(12):1411-1421.

[96] Boucher P, Teasdale N, Courtemanche R, Bard C, Fleury M. Postural stability in diabetic polyneuropathy. Diabetes Care 1995;18(5):638-645.

[97] Bloem BR, Allum JH, Carpenter MG, Honegger F. Is lower leg proprioception essential for triggering human automatic postural responses? Experimental Brain Research 2000;130(3):375-391.

[98] Agrawal Y, Carey J, Della Santina C, Schubert M, Minor LB. Diabetes, Vestibular Dysfunction, and Falls: Analyses From the National Health and Nutrition Examination Survey. Otology & Neurotology 2010;31(9):1445-1450.

[99] Nardone A, Grasso M, Schieppati M. Balance control in peripheral neuropathy: are patients equally unstable under static and dynamic conditions? Gait & Posture 2006;23(3): 364-373.

[100] Krajewski KM, Lewis RA, Fuerst DR, Turansky C, Hinderer SR, Garbern J, Kamholz J, Shy ME. Neurological dysfunction and axonal degeneration in Charcot–Marie–Tooth disease type 1A. Brain 2000;123(7): 1516-1527.

[101] Verhamme C, van Schaik IN, Koelman J, de Haan RJ, de Visser M. The natural history of Charcot–Marie-Tooth type 1A in adults: a 5-year follow-up study. Brain 2009;132;(12):3252-3262.

[102] Uccioli L, Giacomini P, Monticone G, Magrini A, Durols A, Bruno E, Parist L, Di Girolamo S, Menzinger G. Body sway in diabetic neuropathy. Diabetes Care 1995;18(3):339-344.

[103] Oppenheim U, Kohen-Raz R, Alex D, Kohen-Raz A, Azarya M. Postural characteristics of diabetic Neuropathy. Diabetes 1999; 22(2):328-332.

[104] Kanade RV, Van Deursen RW, Harding KG, Price PE. Investigation of standing balance in patients with diabetic neuropathy at different stages of foot complications. Clinical Biomechanics (Bristol, Avon) 2008;23(9): 1183-1191.

[105] Petrofsky JS, Cuneo M, Lee S, Johnson E, Lohman E. Correlation between gait and balance in people with and without Type 2 diabetes in normal and subdued light. Medical Science Monitor 2006; 12(7):CR273-281.

[106] Jáuregui-Renaud K, Sánchez BM, Ibarra-Olmos A, González-Barcena D. Neuro-otologic symptoms in patients with type 2 diabetes mellitus. Diabetes Research and Clinical Practice 2009;84(3):e45-47.

[107] Talbot LA, Musiol RJ, Witham EK, Metter EJ. Falls in young, middle-aged and older community dwelling adults: perceived cause, environmental factors and injury. BMC Public Health 2005; 5:86. doi:10.1186/1471-2458-5-86.

[108] World Health Organization. A global report on falls prevention. Epidemiology of falls. Geneve: World Health Organization; 2007.

[109] Cavanagh PR, Derr JA, Ulbrecht JS, Maser RE, Orchard TJ. Problems with gait and posture in neuropathic patients with insulin- dependent diabetes mellitus. Diabetic Medicine 1992; 9(5):469-474.

[110] DeMott TK, Richardson JK, Thies SB, Ashton-Miller JA. Falls and gait characteristics among older persons with peripheral neuropathy. American Journal of Physical Medicine and Rehabilitation 2007;86(2):125-132.

[111] Lord SR, Lloyd DG, Li SK. Sensori-motor function, gait patterns and falls in community-dwelling women. Age and Ageing 1996; 25(4):292-299.

[112] Richardson JK, Hurvitz EA. Peripheral Neuropathy: A True Risk Factor for Falls. Journals of Gerontology. Series A, Biological Sciences and Medical Sciences 1995;50 (4):M211-215.

[113] Moreland JD, Richardson JA, Goldsmith CH, Clase CM. Muscle weakness and falls in older adults: a systematic review and meta-analysis. Journal of the American Geriatrics Society 2004;52(7):1121-1129.

[114] Kuang TM, Tsai SY, Hsu WM, Cheng CY, Liu JH, Chou P. Visual Impairment and Falls in the Elderly: The Shihpai Eye Study. Journal of the Chinese Medical Association 2008; 71(9): 467-472.

[115] Tinetti ME. Clinical practice. Preventing falls in elderly persons. New England Journal of Medicine 2003:348 (1):42-49.

[116] Huang ES, Karter AJ, Danielson K, Warton EM, Ahmed AT. The Association Between the Number of Prescription Medications and Incident Falls in a Multi-ethnic Population of Adult Type-2 Diabetes Patients: The Diabetes and Aging Study. Journal of General Internal Medicine 2010;25(2):141-146.

[117] Tinetti ME., Medes de Leon CF, Doucette JT, Baker DI. Fear of falling and fall-related efficacy in relationship to functioning among community-living elders. Journal of Gerontology 1994;49 (3):M140–147.

[118] Maki BE, Holliday PJ, Topper AK. Fear of falling and postural performance in the elderly. Journal of Gerontology 1991;46(4): M123-131.

[119] Delbaere K, Crombez G, Vanderstraeten G, Willems T, Cambier D. Fear-related avoidance of activities, falls and physical frailty. A prospective community-based cohort study. Age and Ageing 2004;33(4):368-373.

[120] Richardson JK, Thies SB, DeMott TK, Ashton-Miller JA. Interventions improve gait regularity in patients with peripheral neuropathy while walking on an irregular surface under low light. The Journal of the American Geriatrics Society 2004; 52(4):510–515.

[121] Hausbeck CJ, Strong MJ, Tamkei LS, Leonard WA, Ustinova KI. The effect of additional hand contact on postural stability perturbed by a moving environment. Gait & Posture 2009; 29(3):509-513.

[122] Khaodhiar L, Niemi JB, Earnest R, Lima C, Harry JD, Veves A. Enhancing Sensation in Diabetic Neuropathic Foot With Mechanical Noise. Diabetes Care 2003;26(12): 3280-3283.

[123] Villaume N, Pinsault N. Re-Weighting Of Somatosensory Inputs From The Foot And The Ankle For Controlling Posture During Quiet Standing Following Trunk Extensor Muscles Fatigue. Experimental Brain Research 2007:183(3):323–327.

[124] Maki BE, Perry SD, Norrie RG, McIlroy WE. Effects of facilitation of sensation from plantar foot-surface boundaries on postural stabilization in young and older adults. Journals of Gerontology. Series A, Biological Sciences and Medical Sciences 1999 ; 54(6):M281-287.

[125] Guillebastre B, Calmels P, Rougier PR. Assessment of appropriate ankle-foot orthoses models for patients with Charcot-Marie-Tooth disease. American Journal of Physical Medicine and Rehabilitation 2011;90(8):619-627.

[126] Gardner MM, Robertson MC, Campbell AJ. Exercise in preventing falls and fall related injuries in older people: a review of randomised controlled trials. British Journal of Sports Medicine 2000; 34(1):7–17.

[127] Missaoui B, Thoumie P. How far do patients with sensory ataxia benefit from so-called "proprioceptive rehabilitation"? Neurophysiologie Clinique/Clinical Neurophysiology 2009; 39(4):229-233.

[128] Schneider SH, Amorosa LF, Khachadurian AK, Ruderman NB. Studies on the mechanism of improved glucose control during regular exercise in type 2 (non-insulin-dependent) diabetes. Diabetologia 1984;26(5):355-360.

[129] Hung JW, Liou CW, Wang PW, Yeh SH, Lin LW, Lo SK, Tsai FM. Effect Of 12-Wee K Tai Chi Chuan Exercise On Peripheral Nerve Modulation In Patients With Type 2 Diabetes Mellitus. Journal of Rehabilitation Medicine 2009;41(4): 924–929.

[130] Kruse RL, LeMaster JW, Madsen RW. Fall and Balance Outcomes After an Intervention to Promote Leg Strength, Balance, and Walking in People With Diabetic Peripheral Neuropathy: "Feet First" Randomized Controlled Trial. Physical Therapy 2010;90 (11):1568-1579.

[131] Allet L, Armand S, de Bie RA, Golay A, Monnin D, Aminian K, Staal JB, de Bruin ED. The gait and balance of patients with diabetes can be improved: a randomised controlled trial. Diabetologia 2010;53(3):458–466.

[132] Richardson JK, Sandman D, Vela S. A focused exercise regimen improves clinical measures of balance in patients with peripheral neuropathy. Archives of Physical Medicine and Rehabilitation 2001;82 (2):205-209.

Chapter 6

Predictive Factors for Postherpetic Neuralgia and Recent Pharmacotherapies

Yuko Kanbayashi and Toyoshi Hosokawa

Additional information is available at the end of the chapter

http://dx.doi.org/10.5772/55278

1. Introduction

Postherpetic neuralgia (PHN) is a form of refractory chronic neuralgia that, despite the importance of prevention, currently lacks any effective prophylaxis. The efficacy of live zoster vaccine in preventing PHN was recently reported [1]. However, this vaccine appeared to be of limited use in prophylaxis[2]. PHN has a variety of symptoms and significantly affects patient quality of life [3-12]. Various studies have statistically analyzed predictive factors for PHN [13-23], but neither obvious pathogenesis nor established treatment has been clarified or established. We designed and conducted a study on the premise that statistical identification of significant predictors for PHN would contribute to the establishment of an evidence-based medicine approach to the optimal treatment of PHN. As a result, we reported our paper "Predictive Factors for Postherpetic Neuralgia Using Ordered Logistic Regression Analysis" [24].

In this review, we discuss predictors for PHN based on our results, and further review recent pharmacotherapeutic results.

2. Predictors for PHN

Previous studies have shown that older age, female sex, presence of a prodrome, greater rash severity, and greater acute pain severity are predictors of increased PHN [14-18, 25]. Some other potential predictors (ophthalmic localization, presence of anxiety and depression, presence of allodynia, and serological/virological factors) have also been studied [14, 18]. We conducted a retrospective study to identify significant predictors of PHN that would contribute to the establishment of evidence-based medicine approaches to the optimal treatment of PHN [24].

The participants were 73 patients with herpes zoster who had been treated at the pain clinic of our hospital between January 2008 and June 2010. Variables present at the initial visit were extracted from the clinical records for regression analysis of factors related to the occurrence of PHN. The following scores for response were used: 0 = no PHN after 3 months; 1 = PHN present after 3 months, but absent after 6 months; and 2 = PHN present after 6 months. Multivariate ordered logistic regression analysis was performed to identify predictive factors for PHN. Table 1 shows the clinical characteristics of patients and various factors that could be related to the occurrence of PHN. Multivariate ordered logistic regression analysis identified advanced age and deep pain at the initial visit to our outpatient pain clinic as factors predicting the occurrence of PHN. diabetes mellitus (DM) and pain reduced by bathing also showed high odds ratios, but were not significant predictive factors (Table 2). In conclusion, advanced age and deep pain at first visit were identified as predictive factors for PHN. DM and pain reduced by bathing should also be considered as potential predictors of PHN [24]. To improve patient safety and the likelihood of achieving satisfactory outcomes, prospective studies are needed to establish optimal treatments including pharmacotherapy for PHN. Next section we further review recent pharmacotherapeutic results for PHN.

	(0/1) or (0/1/2), median (range)
Demographics	
Significant zoster-associated pain	35/13/25
Age	8/46/19, 69 (27-90)
Sex	37/36
Complication	
Hypertension	44/29
Angina	69/4
Diabetes mellitus	61/12
Malignant tumor	50/23
Autoimmune disease	68/5
Sleep disorder	36/37
Location	
Trigeminal nerves	58/15
Cervical nerves	58/15
Thoracic nerves	42/31
Lumbar nerves	61/12
Sacral nerves	70/3

http://dx.doi.org/10.5772/55278

	(0/1) or (0/1/2), median (range)
Period of onset, type and extent of pain	
Period before herpes zoster onset (days)	30 (1-3000)
Log (period before herpes zoster onset)	1.477 (0-3.477)
Prodromal rash	39/34
Prodromal pain	34/39
Allodynia	35/38
VAS (mm)	66 (0-100)
Pain reduced when bathing	41/32
Pain (superficial)	35/38
Pain (deep)	38/35
Pain (continuous)	43/30
Pain (breakthrough)	31/42

Binary scales were: female = 0, male = 1 for sex; and absent = 0, present = 1 for others.

The ordered scale was: absent after 3 months = 0, present = 1, and present after 6 months = 2 for significant zoster-associated pain; and <50 years = 0, 51-74 years = 1, ≥75 years = 2 for age.

VAS, visual analog scale

Table 1. Clinical characteristics of 73 patients and various factors that could be related to the occurrence of PHN [24]

Variable	EV	SE	χ^2 value	P	OR	CI of OR	
						Lower 95%	Upper 95%
Age	*1.008*	*0.461*	*4.78*	*0.0288**	*2.740*	*1.110*	*6.761*
Prodromal pain	0.442	0.532	0.69	0.4059	1.556	0.549	4.413
DM	1.123	0.693	2.63	0.1049	3.075	0.791	11.952
Allodynia	0.201	0.630	0.10	0.7489	0.818	0.238	2.808
Pain reduced by bathing	1.221	0.745	2.68	0.1014	3.389	0.787	14.601
Deep pain	*1.446*	*0.682*	*4.49*	*0.0341**	*4.244*	*1.114*	*16.163*
Breakthrough pain	0.687	0.598	1.32	0.2506	1.988	0.616	6.418
Sleep disorder	0.146	0.514	0.08	0.7757	1.158	0.423	3.169

EV, estimated value; SE, standard error; OR, odds ratio; CI, confidence interval; DM, diabetes mellitus

*P<0.05

Table 2. Results of multivariate ordered logistic regression analysis for variables extracted by forward selection with addition of prodromal pain and allodynia [24].

3. Recent pharmacotherapy for PHN

To date, no clear predictors of treatment response have been identified in patients with neuropathic pain, including PHN. Various types of drugs have shown consistent efficacy in randomized clinical trials and meta-analysis [9]. The modes of action and information on dosing, precautions, and adverse events (AEs) for the different drug classes are summarized in Table 3 [9]. Numbers needed to treat (NNTs), numbers needed to harm (NNH) [26, 27] and AEs for the different drugs are shown in Table 4 [28].

Among systemic therapies, tricyclic antidepressants (TCAs), calcium channel α2-δ ligands (gabapentin and pregabalin), and extended-release formulations of morphine and oxycodone show good efficacy in patients with PHN. Current guidelines suggest, perhaps to maximize the benefit-risk ratio, that TCAs should be preferred over opioids, and among TCAs, second-generation TCAs such as nortriptyline, desipramine, and imipramine are preferred over the first-generation agent, amitriptyline [29]. Opioids, specifically oxycodone, morphine, methadone, and tramadol, are also effective against PHN. However, addiction and regulatory issues, coupled with the benign adverse event profile of anticonvulsants, make opioids a secondary choice in PHN [28].

The American Academy of Neurology (AAN; 2004), European Federation of Neurological Societies (NeuPSIG; 2007), and European Federation of Neurological Societies (EFNS; 2010) guidelines all recommend TCAs and pregabalin as first-line oral therapies for patients with PHN [11, 30, 31]. The NeuPSIG and EFNS guidelines also recommend gabapentin as first-line therapy for PHN. The NeuPSIG and EFNS guidelines state that secondary amine TCAs should generally be considered instead of the tertiary amine amitriptyline, due to the superior safety profiles [11, 29, 30].

Japan Society of Pain Clinicians (JSPC; 2011) guidelines recommend TCAs (particularly the secondary amines), calcium channel α2-δ ligands, and extract of cutaneous tissue of rabbits inoculated with vaccinia virus (Neurotropin®) as first-line oral therapies [32].

	Mode of action	Major Adverse- events Precautions Other benefits	Starting dose/maximum dose Titration Duration of adequate trial
Nortriptyline Desipramine	Inhibition of reuptake of serotonin and/or noradrenaline, blockage of sodium channels, anticholinergic	Sedation, ant-cholinergic effects (e.g., dry mouth or urinary retention, weight gain) Cardiac disease , glaucoma, seizure disorder, use of tramadol Improvement of depression and	25 mg at bedtime/150 mg daily Increase by 25 mg every 3-7 day as tolerated 6-8 weeks (at least 2 weeks Maximum tolerated dose)

	Mode of action	Major Adverse- events Precautions Other benefits	Starting dose/maximum dose Titration Duration of adequate trial
		sleep disturbance	
Gabapentin	Decreases release of glutamate, noradrenaline, and substance P, with ligands on α2-δ subunit of voltage-gated calcium channel	Sedation, dizziness, peripheral edema Renal Insufficiency No clinically significant drug interactions	100-300 mg once to three times daily/1200 mg three times daily; reduce if renal function impaired Increase by 100-300 mg three times daily every 1-7 days as Tolerated 4 weeks
Pregabalin	Decreases release of glutamate, noradrenaline, and substance P, with ligands on α2-δ subunit of voltage-gated calcium channel	Sedation, dizziness, Peripheral edema Renal Insufficiency No clinically significant drug interactions, improvement of sleep disturbance and anxiety	50 mg three times daily or 75 mg twice daily/200 mg three times or 300 mg twice daily, reduce if renal function impaired Increase to 300 mg daily after 3-7 days, then by 150 mg daily every 3-7 days, as Tolerated 4 weeks
5% lidocaine patch	Blockage of sodium channels	Local erythema, Rash None No systemic adverse events	1-3 patches/3 patches None 2 weeks
Morphine, oxycodone, methadone, levorphanol	μ-receptor agonism (oxycodone also causes κ-receptor antagonism)	Nausea/ vomiting, constipation, dizziness History of substance abuse, suicide risk, driving impairment Rapid onset of analgesic effect	10-15 mg morphine every 4 h or as needed (equianalgesic doses should be used for other opioids)/no maximum doses After 1-2 weeks convert to long-acting opioids/ transdermal application, use short-acting drug

	Mode of action	Major Adverse- events Precautions Other benefits	Starting dose/maximum dose Titration Duration of adequate trial
			as needed and as tolerated 4-6 weeks

Recommendations are all grading level A = good scientific evidence suggesting that the benefits of the treatment substantially outweigh the potential risks.

Table 3. Recommended first-line treatments for patients with PHN [9]

Drug	NNT (95%CI)	NNH (95%CI)	Specific/Common Adverse Effects
Amitriptyline	1.6 (1.2-2.4) 4.2 (2.13-81.6)	Minor harm: 8 (2.5-22) Major harm: 24 (8-36)	Sedation, dry mouth, tachycardia, constipation, urinary retention, weight gain, prolonged QT interval
Desipramine	1.9 (1.3-3.7)	Minor harm: 4.8 (2.5-36.7) Major harm: 13*	
Nortriptyline	3.7 (2.4-8)	ND	
Gabapentin	4.4 (3.3-6.1)	Minor harm: 4.1 (3.2-5.7) Major harm: 12.3 (7.7-30.2)	Somnolence, dry mouth, weight gain, peripheral edema, ataxia
Pregabalin	4.9 (3.7-7.6)	Minor harm: 4.3 (2.8-9.2) Major harm: ND	Dizziness, somnolence, peripheral edema
Oxycodone	2.5 (1.7-4.4)	Minor harm: 3.6 (2.2-10.2) Major harm: 6.3 (4.2-12.8)	Immune suppression, loss of libido, endocrine dysfunction
Morphine-controlled release or methadone	2.8 (2-4.6)	ND	
Tramadol	4.8 (3.5-6.0)	Minor harm: 7.2* Major harm: 10.8*	Somnolence, constipation, nausea and vomiting, seizures, serotonin syndrome when combined with SSRIs and MAO inhibitors

Values for NNTs and NNHs were adapted from Hempenstall et al. [27] and Wu and Raja [26]. NNTs for amitriptyline were based on studies by Watson et al. [49] and Max et al. [50].

*The 95% confidence interval (CI) could not be determined by Hempenstall et al. [27] or by Wu and Raja [26].

ND, could not be determined by Hempenstall et al [27]; SSRIs, selective serotonin reuptake inhibitors; MAO, monoamine oxidase

Table 4. NNT, NNH, and adverse effects of selected drugs for PHN [28]

http://dx.doi.org/10.5772/55278

3.1. Calcium hannel α2-δ Ligands

Gabapentin and pregabalin suppress the release of excitatory neurotransmitters on binding to the α2-δ subunit of potential-dependent calcium channels in the central nervous system (CNS). Both drugs are structurally similar and share similar mechanisms of action, but pregabalin shows a linear pharmacokinetic profile and strong affinity for the α2-δ subunit. Both drugs have been widely studied in peripheral pain syndromes, although pregabalin has been the focus of most studies in central neuropathic pain syndromes. Only a few drug interactions have been reported for both drugs and the agents are well tolerated, but must be used at lower doses in patients with decreased renal function [9, 32]. The EFNS, AAN, and NeuPSIG guidelines recommend the calcium channel α2-δ ligands gabapentin and/or pregabalin for the treatment of PHN [11, 29-31]. In a meta-analysis, NNTs before 1 patient achieves 50% pain reduction for gabapentin (3 trials, 559 patient episodes) and pregabalin (3 trials, 411 patient episodes) for a 50% reduction in pain were 4.4 and 4.9, respectively [27, 29] (Table 4). Subsequent Cochrane reviews for both drugs calculated NNTs of 7.5 for gabapentin [29, 33] and 3.9 for pregabalin 600 mg [29, 34]. Gabapentin and pregabalin are effective and are the most commonly prescribed drugs in PHN because of their efficacy and benign AEs profile.

3.1.1. Pregabalin

Pregabalin is a 3-isobutyl derivative of gamma-amino butyric acid (GABA) with anti-convulsant, anti-epileptic, anxiolytic, and analgesic activities. Although the exact mechanisms of action are unclear, pregabalin selectively binds to α2-δ subunits of presynaptic voltage-dependent calcium channels located in the CNS. Binding of pregabalin to α2-δ subunits of presynaptic voltage-dependent calcium channels prevents calcium influx and the subsequent calcium-dependent release of various neurotransmitters, including glutamate, noradrenaline, serotonin (5-Hydroxytryptamine: 5-HT), dopamine, and substance P, from the presynaptic nerve terminals of hyperexcited neurons; synaptic transmission is inhibited and neuronal excitability is diminished. Pregabalin does not bind directly to GABA-A or GABA-B receptors and does not alter GABA uptake or degradation [35].

Pregabalin has also been associated with dose-related risks of somnolence (5-14%), dizziness (7-28%), and peripheral edema (6-16%) [29, 32, 34]. At a higher dose (600 mg/day), pregabalin has been associated with weight gain (9%), asthenia (9%), dry mouth (6%), and vertigo (5%) [28, 29, 36]. Discontinuations due to these AEs were ≤1% in patients treated with pregabalin at 150 mg/day and 4-15% in patients receiving a 600-mg/day dose. Serious AEs were reported in 2-5% of patients treated with pregabalin at 150, 300, and 600 mg/day, compared with 3% in those assigned to receive a placebo [29, 36]. Symptoms including insomnia, nausea, headache, and diarrhea were reported by some patients following abrupt withdrawal of pregabalin. Pregabalin should therefore be tapered gradually over a minimum of 1 week rather than discontinued abruptly. Weight gain noted in clinical trials of pregabalin was not limited to patients with peripheral edema. Weight gain was related to dose and duration of exposure to pregabalin, but did not appear to be associated with sex, age, or baseline body-mass index. A higher incidence of weight gain and peripheral edema were noted in patients taking both pregabalin and a thiazolidinedione, compared with patients taking either agent alone. As a result, care should be taken when co-administering pregabalin and one of these agents [37].

JSPC guidelines recommend beginning pregabalin treatment at 75 mg/day once before bed, 150 mg/day as two doses after breakfast and supper, or 150 mg/day as three doses after each meal. Even when renal function is normal, consider a very low dose only just before bed, such as 25 mg/day once before bed, for elderly patients, patients of low body weight, and others prone to AEs [32].

3.1.2. Gabapentin

Gabapentin is a synthetic analogue of the neurotransmitter GABA with anticonvulsant activity. Although the exact mechanisms of action are unknown, gabapentin appears to inhibit excitatory neuron activity. This agent also exhibits analgesic properties [35].

In clinical trials, the most frequent AEs observed with gabapentin were somnolence (16%), dizziness (21%), and peripheral edema (8%) [33]. Twelve percent of patients discontinued gabapentin owing to AEs, compared with 8% who discontinued placebo. Serious AEs with gabapentin and placebo occurred in 4% and 3% of patients, respectively [29].

3.2. Opioids

Opioid analgesics are agonists at presynaptic and postsynaptic opioid receptors. Opioids offer comparable analgesic efficacy to TCAs. Concerns about long-term AEs, such as immunological changes, physical dependency, and misuse or abuse, can limit the use of strong opioids in patients with neuropathic non-cancer-related pain [9].

The place of opioids and tramadol in guidelines for the management of PHN has evolved over time. In the 2004 AAN guidelines, extended-release formulations of oxycodone and morphine were recommended as first-line agents. Guidelines issued by the NeuPSIG (2007) and EFNS (2010) recommend strong opioids and tramadol as second-line therapy, not because of new data on efficacy, but perhaps reflecting concerns about the risks of AEs and abuse [29].

Extended-release formulations of oxycodone [38] and morphine, as well as methadone [39], have shown efficacy in patients with PHN. The NNT for a 50% reduction in pain were 2.5 for oxycodone and 2.8 for morphine or methadone, compared with an NNT of 3.7 for the TCA nortriptyline (Table 4). In a placebo-controlled, active comparator-controlled crossover trial, the majority of patients (53%) preferred the opioids morphine or methadone over TCAs. Opioids tended to provide greater pain relief, although the difference was not significant [40]. A meta-analysis of the 2 trials evaluating oxycodone, morphine and methadone calculated an NNT for opioids of 2.7 [27]. Tramadol has proven less effective than strong opioids. In a randomized controlled trial, tramadol was not significantly better than placebo on a 5-point verbal scale or on measures of quality of life [40]. An analysis of this trial calculated an NNT of 4.8 [27]. Oxycodone, morphine, and methadone were associated with typical opioid-related AEs, including nausea, diarrhea, and constipation [38, 39]. Tramadol was better tolerated, but less effective [40].

In the JSPC guideline, although multiple clinical studies have demonstrated the analgesic effects of opioid analgesics (narcotics for medical use) in patients with neuropathic pain, opioids are generally recommended as second- or third-line treatment for several reasons. First, opioid analgesics have a high incidence of associated AEs that may persist over the entire course of treatment. Second, the lack of any systematic investigation into the long-term safety of opioid analgesics means that the opioid analgesics may not be fundamentally safer than other drug options. Third, opioid analgesics may cause hyperalgesia. This effect, if present, would adversely modify the risk/benefit profile of long-term treatment in neuropathic pain patients. Finally, opioid abuse and addiction are substantial problems [32].

3.2.1. Morphine

The sulfate salt of morphine is an opiate alkaloid isolated from the plant Papaver somniferum and produced synthetically. Morphine binds to and activates specific opiate receptors (δ, μ and κ), each of which are involved in controlling different brain functions. In the CNS and gastrointestinal system, this agent exerts widespread effects including analgesia, anxiolysis, euphoria, sedation, respiratory depression, and smooth muscle contraction in the gastrointestinal system.

A sustained-release tablet formulation contains the sulfate salt of the opiate alkaloid morphine to provide analgesic activity. Morphine binds to and activates μ-opioid receptors in the CNS, thereby mimicking the effects of endogenous opioids. Binding of morphine to opioid receptors stimulates exchange of guanosine 5'-triphosphate for guanosine 5'-diphosphate, inhibits adenylate cyclase, and decreases intracellular cyclic adenosine monophosphate. This inhibits the release of various nociceptive neurotransmitters, such as substance P, GABA, dopamine, acetylcholine, noradrenaline, vasopressin, and somatostatin. In addition, morphine closes N-type voltage-gated calcium channels and opens calcium-dependent inwardly rectifying potassium channels, causing hyperpolarization of neuronal membranes and reductions in neuronal excitability, with subsequent analgesia and sedation [35].

3.2.2. Oxycodone hydrochloride

The hydrochloride salt of oxycodone is a methylether of oxymorphone and a semisynthetic opioid agonist with analgesic and antitussive properties. Oxycodone binds to μ-receptors in the CNS, thereby mimicking the effects of endogenous opiates as well as morphine. In addition to analgesia and a depressive effect on the cough center in the medulla, this agent may cause euphoria, anxiolysis, miosis, sedation, physical dependence, constipation, and respiratory depression, depending on dosage and variations in individual metabolism [35].

3.2.3. Tramadol

A synthetic codeine analogue, tramadol has central analgesic properties with effects similar to opioids, such as morphine and codeine, acting on specific opioid receptors. Used as a narcotic analgesic for severe pain, this agent can be addictive. Tramadol is used to treat moderate-to-severe pain in adults, and binds to opioid receptors in the CNS[41]. Tramadol also weakly inhibits noradrenaline and 5-HT reuptake and can therefore interact with serotonergic drugs (selective noradrenaline reuptake inhibitors [SNRIs] and selective serotonin reuptake inhibitors [SSRIs]), causing serotonin syndrome, although this risk seems to be low in clinical practice [9].

3.3. TCAs

Clinical data support the efficacy of TCAs for PHN. In a 2005 meta-analysis of 4 clinical trials (248 patient episodes), the NNT for 1 patient to achieve a 50% reduction in pain with the TCAs amitriptyline, nortriptyline, and desipramine was 2.6 [27]. A 2007 Cochrane review of 4 clinical trials (244 patients) calculated an NNT of 2.7 [41]. Although effective, TCAs have been associated with significant systemic AEs, most notably anticholinergic AEs [43, 44], and have been associated with cardiotoxicity [45-47]. Electrocardiography (ECG) before the start of treatment is mandatory and careful dose titration is needed [9]. Individual trials of amitriptyline and desipramine in patients with PHN suggest that the second-generation TCA desipramine produces fewer anticholinergic side effects than amitriptyline [48, 49].

3.3.1. Amitriptyline hydrochloride

The hydrochloride salt of the tricyclic dibenzocycloheptadiene amitriptyline with antidepressant and antinociceptive activities. Amitriptyline hydrochloride is the hydrochloride salt of the tricyclic dibenzocycloheptadiene amitriptyline, and shows antidepressant and antinociceptive activities. Amitriptyline inhibits the re-uptake of noradrenaline and serotonin by the presynaptic neuronal membrane in the CNS, thereby increasing synaptic concentrations of noradrenaline and serotonin. Due to constant stimulation of these receptors, amitriptyline may produce a downregulation of adrenergic and serotonin receptors, which may contribute to the antidepressant activity. In the CNS, the antinociceptive activity of this agent may involve high-affinity binding to and inhibition of N-methyl-D-aspartate (NMDA) receptors and/or enhancement of the action of serotonin at the spinal terminals of an opioid-mediated intrinsic analgesia system [35].

Amitriptyline has an NNT of 2.2 for PHN, but the AEs, lack of recommendations for use in the elderly, and small sample sizes of studies have relegated this agent behind antiepileptics for certain PHN cases [30, 42, 50, 51]. Nortriptyline, maprotiline, and desipramine have also proven effective, but less so than amitriptyline.

3.3.2. Nortriptyline

A TCA used for short-term treatment of various forms of depression, nortriptyline blocks the noradrenaline presynaptic receptors, thereby blocking reuptake of this neurotransmitter and raising concentrations in the synaptic cleft in the CNS. Nortriptyline also binds to α-adrenergic, histaminergic and cholinergic receptors. Long-term treatment with nortriptyline produces downregulation of adrenergic receptors due to increased stimulation of these receptors [41].

3.4. Selective serotonin and noradrenaline reuptake inhibitors

Patients who are unable to tolerate TCAs may do better with selective serotonin and noradrenaline reuptake inhibitors, such as duloxetine or venlafaxine. Although less effective than

TCAs, the selective 5-HT and noradrenaline reuptake inhibitors (SSNRIs) offer efficacy for both pain and depression with fewer AEs. SSRIs effectively relieve depression symptoms but they do not specifically relieve neuropathic pain. Nevertheless, some patients with chronic pain due to PHN will experience clinical depression, and the use of SSRIs can be useful for the management of depressive symptoms [5].

SNRIs are safer and easier to use than TCAs and represent a better option for patients with heart disease. The mechanism of SNRI analgesia is likely associated with activation of the descending inhibitory system of pain.

3.4.1. *Paroxetine hydrochloride*

The hydrochloride salt form of paroxetine is a phenylpiperidine derivative and a SSRI with antidepressant and anxiolytic properties. Paroxetine binds to the pre-synaptic serotonin transporter complex, resulting in negative allosteric modulation of the complex and thereby blocking reuptake of serotonin by the pre-synaptic transporter. Inhibition of serotonin recycling enhances serotonergic function through serotonin accumulation in the synaptic cleft, resulting in long-term desensitization and downregulation of 5-HT receptors and leading to symptomatic relief of depressive illness [35].

3.4.2. *Duloxetine hydrochloride*

The hydrochloride salt of duloxetine is a fluoxetine derivative belonging to the class of SSNRIs and exhibiting antidepressant activity. Duloxetine selectively prevents reuptake of 5-HT and noradrenaline via transporter complexes on the pre-synaptic membrane, thereby increasing the levels of these neurotransmitters within the synaptic cleft. As a result, this agent potentiates serotonergic and noradrenergic activities in the CNS, alleviating depression and neuropathic sensations such as pain and tingling. Furthermore, duloxetine does not show significant affinity for dopaminergic, adrenergic, cholinergic, histaminergic, opioid, glutamatergic, or GABAergic receptors [35].

Duloxetine is recommended for painful diabetic neuropathies [11, 29, 30], but not for PHN; little clinical trial data has been accumulated supporting use in PHN. SNRIs are also associated with a number of systemic AEs, including nausea, vomiting, somnolence, anorexia, constipation, dizziness, fatigue, insomnia, increased sweating, and dry mouth [52-54].

3.5. Other oral therapies

Several other oral agents have been investigated in the treatment of PHN. Specifically, the NMDA antagonists dextromethorphan and memantine [55, 56] and the benzodiazepine lorazepam [56] have not shown good efficacy in clinical trials.

In treatment guidelines, therapies described as lacking sufficient evidence of efficacy include anticonvulsants that target sodium channels (carbamazepine and oxcarbazepine), other anticonvulsants (lamotrigine, topiramate, and valproic acid), other antidepressants (bupropion, citalopram, paroxetine), and the oral lidocaine analog, mexiletine [11, 30, 31]. For other neuropathic pain syndromes, mexiletine has only shown efficacy at doses that produce systemic AEs, including proarrhythmic effects [43]. This suggests that the benefits of sodium channel antagonism for PHN may be better achieved via local lidocaine administration.

JSPC guidelines also recommend extract of cutaneous tissue from rabbits inoculated with vaccinia virus (Neurotropin®) as a first-line oral therapy[32].

3.5.1. *Carbamazepine*

Carbamazepine is a tricyclic compound chemically related to TCAs with anticonvulsant and analgesic properties. This agent exerts anticonvulsant activity by reducing polysynaptic responses and blocking post-tetanic potentiation. The analgesic activity is not understood, but carbamazepine is commonly used to treat pain associated with trigeminal neuralgia [35].

3.5.2. *Valproic acid*

Valproic acid is a synthetic derivative of propylpentanoic acid with antiepileptic properties and potential antineoplastic and antiangiogenesis activities. In epilepsy, valproic acid appears to act by increasing concentrations of GABA in the brain. The antitumor and antiangiogenesis activities of this agent may be related to the inhibition of histone deacetylases and nitric oxide synthase, resulting in the inhibition of nitric oxide synthesis [35].

3.5.3. *Extract of cutaneous tissue from rabbits inoculated with vaccinia virus*

Extract of cutaneous tissue from rabbits inoculated with vaccinia virus (Neurotropin®) has been shown to exert analgesic effects in a Japanese clinical study in PHN as one type of neuropathic pain. Producing no serious AEs, the drug product was very well tolerated, in addition to conferring analgesic effects. The drug product has been clinically used in patients 20 years old and older and is very safe [32, 57, 58].

3.5.4. *Antiarrhythmics (mexiletine)*

Mexiletine hydrochloride is a class 1B antiarrhythmic, and works by blocking sodium channels. A local anesthetic and antiarrhythmic (Class IB) agent structurally related to lidocaine, mexiletine exerts antiarrhythmic effects by inhibiting the inward sodium current in cardiac cells, thus reducing the rate of increase in the cardiac action potential (phase 0) and decreasing automaticity in Purkinje fibers. This slows nerve impulses in the heart and stabilizes the heartbeat. The anesthetic activity is due to the ability of mexiletine to block sodium influx in peripheral nerves, thereby reducing the rate and intensity of pain impulses reaching the CNS [41].

3.5.5. *Lidocaine patch 5%*

Lidocaine relieves pain through non-specific blockage of sodium channels on ectopic peripheral afferent fibers without causing numbness of the treated skin. Topical application without

http://dx.doi.org/10.5772/55278

a relevant systemic absorption offers a good benefit-to-risk ratio only with local AEs, such as erythema or rash [9].

The transdermal patch contains a 5% aqueous base solution of the synthetic amide-type anesthetic lidocaine with analgesic activity. Upon topical application and transdermal delivery, the active ingredient lidocaine binds to and blocks voltage-gated sodium channels in the neuronal cell membrane; lidocaine-mediated stabilization of neuronal membranes inhibits the initiation and conduction of nerve impulses and produces reversible local anesthesia [34]. The lidocaine 5% patch is recommended as first-line therapy in the AAN [31], NeuPSIG [30], and EFNS [11] guidelines [29].

3.6. Combination therapy

In clinical practice, a combination of two or more drugs is often needed to achieve satisfactory pain relief, although few trials have been conducted to support this clinical observation. However, combination therapy with gabapentin or pregabalin and extended-release morphine in patients with PHN achieved higher pain relief with lower doses compared to administration of one drug alone. These results have also been confirmed for the combination of nortriptyline and gabapentin as well as for pregabalin and topical lidocaine in patients with PHN. Taken together, these results substantiate the usefulness of combination therapies in patients with PHN [9].

4. Conclusion

Neither obvious pathogenesis nor an established treatment have been clarified or established for PHN. Our study indicated that advanced age and deep pain at the first visit were shown to be predictive factors for PHN. DM and pain reduced by bathing should also be considered as potential predictors of PHN. We further reviewed recent pharmacotherapeutic results for PHN. To improve patient safety and the likelihood of achieving satisfactory outcomes, prospective studies are needed to establish optimal treatments including pharmacotherapy for PHN.

Author details

Yuko Kanbayashi[1,2*] and Toyoshi Hosokawa[2,3,4]

*Address all correspondence to: ykokanba@koto.kpu-m.ac.jp

1 Department of Hospital Pharmacy, Kyoto Prefectural University of Medicine, Graduate School of Medical Science, Kyoto, Japan

2 Pain Treatment & Palliative Care Unit, University Hospital, Kyoto Prefectural University of Medicine, Graduate School of Medical Science, Kyoto, Japan

3 Department of Anaesthesiology, Kyoto Prefectural University of Medicine, Graduate School of Medical Science, Kyoto, Japan

4 Pain Management & Palliative Care Medicine, Kyoto Prefectural University of Medicine, Graduate School of Medical Science, Kyoto, Japan

References

[1] Gilden D. Efficacy of live zoster vaccine in preventing zoster and postherpetic neuralgia J Intern Med 2011; 269: 496-506.

[2] Li Q, Chen N, Yang J, Zhou M, Zhou D, Zhang Q, He L. Antiviral treatment for preventing postherpetic neuralgia. Cochrane Database Syst Rev 2009; 2. CD006866.

[3] Schmader KE. Epidemiology and impact on quality of life of postherpetic neuralgia and painful diabetic neuropathy. Clin J Pain 2002; 18: 350-354.

[4] Dworkin RH, Portenoy RK. Pain and its persistence in herpes zoster. Pain 1996; 67: 241-251.

[5] Sampathkumar P, Drage LA, Martin DP. Herpes zoster (shingles) and postherpetic neuralgia. Mayo Clin Proc. 2009; 84: 274-280.

[6] Johnson RW. Herpes zoster and postherpetic neuralgia. Expert Rev Vaccines 2010; 9: 21-26.

[7] McElhaney JE. Herpes zoster: a common disease that can have a devastating impact on patients' quality of life. Expert Rev Vaccines 2010; 9: 27-30.

[8] Johnson RW, McElhaney J. Postherpetic neuralgia in the elderly. J Int J Clin Pract 2009; 63: 1386-1391.

[9] Baron R, Binder A, Wasner G. Neuropathic pain: diagnosis, pathophysiological mechanisms, and treatment. Lancet Neurol 2010; 9: 807-819.

[10] Whitley RJ, Volpi A, McKendrick M, Wijck A, Oaklander AL. Management of herpes zoster and post-herpetic neuralgia now and in the future. J Clin Virol 2010; 48:S20-S28.

[11] Attal N, Cruccu G, Baron R, Haanpää M, Hansson P, Jensen TS, Nurmikko T; European Federation of Neurological Societies. EFNS guidelines on the pharmacological treatment of neuropathic pain: 2010 revision. Eur J Neurol 2010; 17: 1113-e88.

[12] Doth AH, Hansson PT, Jensen MP, Taylor RS. The burden of neuropathic pain: a systematic review and meta-analysis of health utilities. Pain 2010; 149: 338-344.

[13] Jung BF, Johnson RW, Griffin DR, Dworkin RH. Risk factors for postherpetic neuralgia in patients with herpes zoster. Neurology 2004; 62: 1545-1551.

[14] Dworkin RH, Nagasako EM, Johnson RW, Griffin DR. Acute pain in herpes zoster: the famciclovir database project. Pain 2001; 94: 113-119.

[15] Kurokawa I, Kumano K, Murakawa K. Hyogo Prefectural PHN Study Group. Clinical correlates of prolonged pain in Japanese patients with acute herpes zoster. J Int Med Res 2002; 30: 56-65.

[16] Scott FT, Leedham-Green ME, Barrett-Muir WY, Hawrami K, Gallagher WJ, Johnson R, Breuer J. A study of shingles and the development of postherpetic neuralgia in East London. J Med Virol 2003; 70: S24-S30.

[17] Nithyanandam S, Dabir S, Stephen J, Joseph M. Eruption severity and characteristics in herpes zoster ophthalmicus: correlation with visual outcome, ocular complications, and postherpetic neuralgia. Int J Dermatol 2009; 48: 484-487.

[18] Opstelten W, Zuithoff NP, van Essen GA, van Loon AM, van Wijck AJ, Kalkman CJ, Verheij TJ, Moons KG. Predicting postherpetic neuralgia in elderly primary care patients with herpes zoster: prospective prognostic study. Pain 2007; 132: S52-S59.

[19] Parruti G, Tontodonati M, Rebuzzi C, Polilli E, Sozio F, Consorte A, Agostinone A, Di Masi F, Congedo G, D'Antonio D, Granchelli C, D'Amario C, Carunchio C, Pippa L, Manzoli L, Volpi A; VZV Pain Study Group. Predictors of pain intensity and persistence in a prospective Italian cohort of patients with herpes zoster: relevance of smoking, trauma and antiviral therapy. BMC Med 2010; 8: 58.

[20] Volpi A, Gatti A, Pica F, Bellino S, Marsella LT, Sabato AF. Clinical and psychosocial correlates of post-herpetic neuralgia. J Med Virol 2008; 80: 1646-1652.

[21] McKendrick MW, Ogan P, Care CC. A 9 year follow up of post herpetic neuralgia and predisposing factors in elderly patients following herpes zoster. J Infect 2009; 59: 416-420.

[22] Drolet M, Brisson M, Schmader K, Levin M, Johnson R, Oxman M, Patrick D, Camden S, Mansi JA. Predictors of postherpetic neuralgia among patients with herpes zoster: a prospective study. J Pain 2010; 11: 1211-1221.

[23] Mick G, Gallais JL, Simon F, Pinchinat S, Bloch K, Beillat M, Serradell L, Derrough T. Burden of herpes zoster and postherpetic neuralgia: Incidence, proportion, and associated costs in the French population aged 50 or over. Rev Epidemiol Sante Publique 2010; 58: 393-401.

[24] Kanbayashi Y, Onishi K, Fukazawa K, Okamoto K, Ueno H, Takagi T, Hosokawa T. Predictive Factors for Postherpetic Neuralgia Using Ordered Logistic Regression Analysis. Clin J Pain 2011, in press.

[25] Johnson RW. Zoster-associated pain: what is known, who is at risk and how can it be managed? Herpes 2007; 14: 30-34.

[26] Wu CL, Raja SN. An update on the treatment of postherpetic neuralgia. J Pain 2008; 9: S19-30.

[27] Hempenstall K, Nurmikko TJ, Johnson RW, A'Hern RP, Rice AS. Analgesic therapy in postherpetic neuralgia: a quantitative systematic review. PLoS Med 2005; 2: e164.

[28] Benzon HT, Chekka K, Darnule A, Chung B, Wille O, Malik K. Evidence-based case report: the prevention and management of postherpetic neuralgia with emphasis on interventional procedures. Reg Anesth Pain Med 2009; 34: 514-21.

[29] Argoff CE. Review of current guidelines on the care of postherpetic neuralgia. Postgrad Med 2011; 123: 134-142.

[30] Dworkin RH, O'Connor AB, Backonja M, Farrar JT, Finnerup NB, Jensen TS, Kalso EA, Loeser JD, Miaskowski C, Nurmikko TJ, Portenoy RK, Rice AS, Stacey BR, Treede RD, Turk DC, Wallace MS. Pharmacologic management of neuropathic pain: evidence-based recommendations. Pain 2007; 132: 237-251.

[31] Dubinsky RM, Kabbani H, El-Chami Z, Boutwell C, Ali H; Quality Standards Subcommittee of the American Academy of Neurology. Practice parameter: treatment of postherpetic neuralgia: an evidence-based report of the Quality Standards Subcommittee of the American Academy of Neurology. Neurology. 2004; 63: 959-965.

[32] The Committee for the Guidelines for the Pharmacologic Management of Neuropathic Pain of JSPC. Guidelines for the Pharmacologic Management of Neuropathic Pain. Tokyo: Shinko Trading; 2011.

[33] Moore RA, Wiffen PJ, Derry S, McQuay HJ. Gabapentin for chronic neuropathic pain and fibromyalgia in adults. Cochrane Database Syst Rev 2011; 3: CD007938.

[34] Moore RA, Straube S, Wiffen PJ, Derry S, McQuay HJ. Pregabalin for acute and chronic pain in adults. Cochrane Database Syst Rev 2009; 3: CD007076.

[35] National Cancer Institute. National Cancer Institute of the National Institutes of Health (NIH). Cancer topics, In: Cancer Drug Information. 2012 http://www.cancer.gov/drugdictionary (accessed 12 August).

[36] Freeman R, Durso-Decruz E, Emir B. Efficacy, safety, and tolerability of pregabalin treatment for painful diabetic peripheral neuropathy: findings from seven randomized, controlled trials across a range of doses. Diabetes Care 2008; 31: 1448-1454.

[37] Cappuzzo KA. Treatment of postherpetic neuralgia: focus on pregabalin. Clin Interv Aging 2009; 4: 17-23.

[38] Watson CP, Babul N. Efficacy of oxycodone in neuropathic pain: a randomized trial in postherpetic neuralgia. Neurology 1998; 50: 1837-1841.

[39] Raja SN, Haythornthwaite JA, Pappagallo M, Clark MR, Travison TG, Sabeen S, Royall RM, Max MB. Opioids versus antidepressants in postherpetic neuralgia: a randomized, placebo-controlled trial. Neurology 2002; 59: 1015-1021.

[40] Boureau F, Legallicier P, Kabir-Ahmadi M. Tramadol in post-herpetic neuralgia: a randomized, double-blind, placebo-controlled trial. Pain 2003; 104: 323–331.

[41] National Cancer Institute. National Cancer Institute of the National Institutes of Health (NIH). NCI Thesaurus. 2012 http://ncit.nci.nih.gov/ncitbrowser/pages/home.jsf (accessed 12 August).

[42] Saarto T, Wiffen PJ. Antidepressants for neuropathic pain. Cochrane Database Syst Rev 2007; 4: CD005454.

[43] Finnerup NB, Otto M, McQuay HJ, Jensen TS, Sindrup SH. Algorithm for neuropathic pain treatment: an evidence based proposal. Pain 2005; 118: 289-305.

[44] Sindrup SH, Otto M, Finnerup NB, Jensen TS. Antidepressants in the treatment of neuropathic pain. Basic Clin Pharmacol Toxicol 2005; 96: 399-409.

[45] Cohen HW, Gibson G, Alderman MH. Excess risk of myocardial infarction in patients treated with antidepressant medications: association with use of tricyclic agents. Am J Med 2000; 108: 2-8.

[46] Ray WA, Meredith S, Thapa PB, Hall K, Murray KT. Cyclic antidepressants and the risk of sudden cardiac death. Clin Pharmacol Ther 2004; 75: 234-241.

[47] Tata LJ, West J, Smith C, Farrington P, Card T, Smeeth L, Hubbard R. General population based study of the impact of tricyclic and selective serotonin reuptake inhibitor antidepressants on the risk of acute myocardial infarction. Heart 2005; 91: 465-471.

[48] Max MB, Lynch SA, Muir J, Shoaf SE, Smoller B, Dubner R. Effects of desipramine, amitriptyline, and fluoxetine on pain in diabetic neuropathy. N Engl J Med 1992; 326: 1250-1256.

[49] Watson CP, Vernich L, Chipman M, Reed K. Nortriptyline versus amitriptyline in postherpetic neuralgia: a randomized trial. Neurology 1998; 51: 1166-1171.

[50] Watson CP, Evans RJ, Reed K, Merskey H, Goldsmith I, Warsh J. Amitriptyline versus placebo in postherpetic neuralgia. Neurology 1982; 32: 671-673.

[51] Max MB, Schafer SC, Culnane M, Smoller B, Dubner R, Gracely RH. Amitriptyline, but not lorazepam, relieves postherpetic neuralgia. Neurology 1988; 38: 1427-1432.

[52] Lunn MP, Hughes RA, Wiffen PJ. Duloxetine for treating painful neuropathy or chronic pain. Cochrane Database Syst Rev 2009; 4: CD007115.

[53] Raskin J, Smith TR, Wong K, Pritchett YL, D'Souza DN, Iyengar S, Wernicke JF. Duloxetine versus routine care in the long-term management of diabetic peripheral neuropathic pain. J Palliat Med 2006; 9: 29-40.

[54] Wernicke JF, Pritchett YL, D'Souza DN, Waninger A, Tran P, Iyengar S, Raskin J. A randomized controlled trial of duloxetine in diabetic peripheral neuropathic pain. Neurology 2006; 67: 1411-1420.

[55] Sang CN, Booher S, Gilron I, Parada S, Max MB. Dextromethorphan and memantine in painful diabetic neuropathy and postherpetic neuralgia: efficacy and dose-response trials. Anesthesiology 2002; 96: 1053-1061.

[56] Wallace MS, Rowbotham MC, Katz NP, Dworkin RH, Dotson RM, Galer BS, Rauck RL, Backonja MM, Quessy SN, Meisner PD. A randomized, double-blind, placebo-controlled trial of a glycine antagonist in neuropathic pain. Neurology 2002; 59: 1694-1700.

[57] Kawashiri T, Egashira N, Watanabe H, Ikegami Y, Hirakawa S, Mihara Y, Yano T, Ikesue H, Oishi R. Prevention of oxaliplatin-induced mechanical allodynia and neurodegeneration by neurotropin in the rat model. Eur J Pain. 2011; 15:344-50.

[58] Kudo T, Kushikata T, Kudo M, Kudo T, Hirota K. Antinociceptive effects of neurotropin in a rat model of central neuropathic pain: DSP-4 induced noradrenergic lesion. Neurosci Lett. 2011; 503:20-2.